www.wadsworth.com

wadsworth.com is the World Wide Web site for Wadsworth and is your direct source to dozens of online resources.

At *wadsworth.com* you can find out about supplements, demonstration software, and student resources. You can also send email to many of our authors and preview new publications and exciting new technologies.

wadsworth.com
Changing the way the world learns®

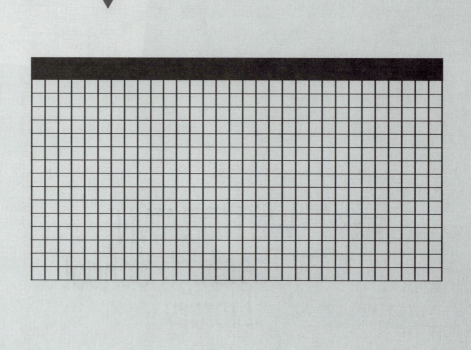

Badminton Today

Second ▲ Edition

Sunny Kim

Mike Walker

Series Editor
Bob O'Connor

WADSWORTH ™

THOMSON LEARNING

Australia • Canada • Mexico • Singapore • Spain • United Kingdom • United States

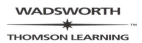

WADSWORTH
THOMSON LEARNING

Publisher: Peter Marshall
Associate Editor: April Lemons
Assistant Editor: John Boyd
Editorial Assistant: Andrea Kesterke
Marketing Manager: Joanne Terhaar
Marketing Assistant: Justine Ferguson
Advertising Project Manager: Brian Chaffee
Project Manager: Sandra Craig

Print/Media Buyer: Robert King
Permissions Editor: Stephanie Keough-Hedges
Production and Composition: Ash Street Typecrafters, Inc.
Text and Cover Designer: Harry Voigt
Copy Editor: Laura Larson
Cover Image: VCG / FPG International
Printer: The Mazer Corporation

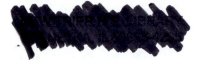

Wadsworth/Thomson Learning
10 Davis Drive
Belmont, CA 94002-3098
USA

For more information about our products, contact us:
Thompson Learning Academic Resource Center
1-800-423-0563
http://www.wadsworth.com

International Headquarters
Thomson Learning
International Division
290 Harbor Drive, 2nd Floor
Stamford, CT 06902-7477
USA

UK/Europe/Middle East/South Africa
Thomson Learning
Berkshire House
168-173 High Holborn
London WC1V 7AA
United Kingdom

Asia
Thomson Learning
60 Albert Street, #15-01
Albert Complex
Singapore 189969

Canada
Nelson Thomson Learning
1120 Birchmount Road
Toronto, Ontario M1K 5G4
Canada

Library of Congress Cataloging-in-Publication Data

Kim, Sunny.
   Badminton today / Sunny Kim, Mike Walker.—2nd ed.
     p. cm.
   Rev. ed. of: Badminton today / Tariq Wadood, Karlyne Tan.
     c1990.
   Includes index.
   ISBN 0-534-55233-1
   1. Badminton (Game) I. Walker, Mike (Michael E. D.)
     II. Wadood, Tariq. Badminton today. III. Title.

   GV1007 .K55 2001
   796.345—dc21

                        2001024869

Contents

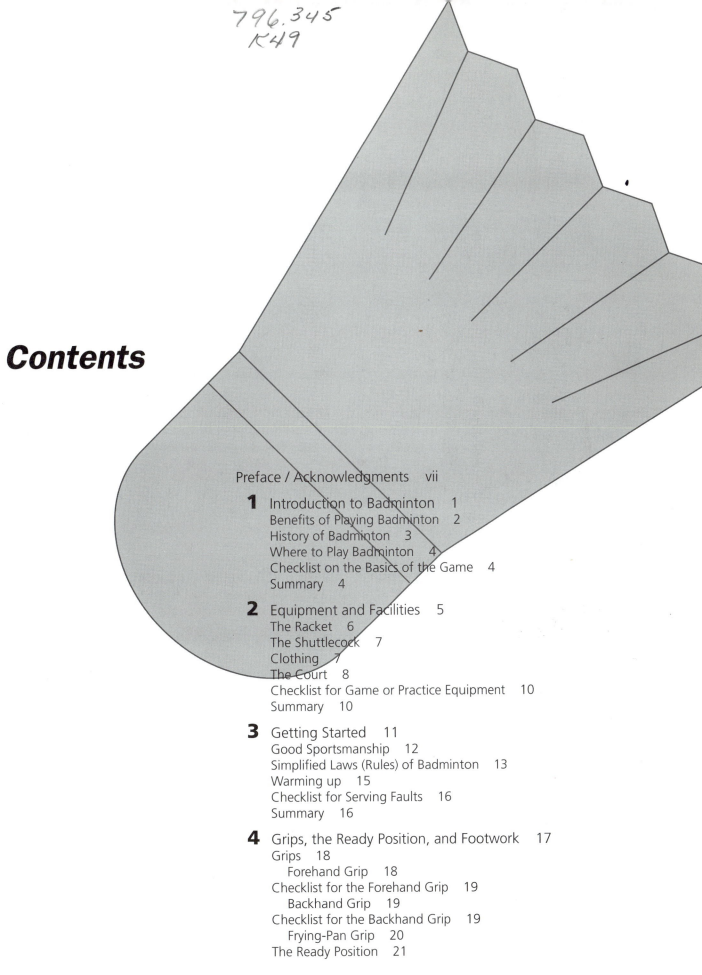

Preface

Badminton has long had stature as a major sport in much of the world. Today, with badminton being an Olympic sport, its popularity is rising rapidly in the United States. With the rapid increase in the popularity of the sport we thought that it was necessary to develop a book that will allow everyone to learn the sport correctly and to enjoy it more.

We have worked diligently to give you the basics in every area—from the rules and courtesies of the game to the strokes and strategies. The book allows the player to progress from beginning, to intermediate, and to the advanced levels of play.

The publishers have spared no expense in allowing us to show every aspect of the game in photographs and drawings so that you readers can get the most from our presentation. We have explained the details of the game and have emphasized them in various checklists in each chapter. These checklists will help you to follow a skill simply so you can do it correctly even if you are a beginning level player.

We hope you will enjoy reading the book and playing the game as much as we have enjoyed writing it for you. Have fun!

Acknowledgments

The development of this text could not have progressed without the helpful criticisms and suggestions from our colleagues. A special thanks to Christina Kranzler and David Hanover for the photography.

The authors gratefully acknowledge the following:

Reviewers

William Barfield
College of Charleston

Susan Whitlock
Kennesaw State University

Tom Peterson
State University of West Georgia

Ronnie Akers
State University of West Georgia

About the Authors

Mike Walker

Mike Walker has been a national champion at different levels more than 40 times. He has also been a Thomas Cup team member. As a teacher he has developed programs to increase the skill level of players at every level. As Chairman of the Coaches Committee for USA Badminton he is currently working with others to develop an even more effective coaching system. He has coached the Uber Cup team as well as many other high level teams.

Sunny Kim

Sunny Kim was the 1988 United States Collegiate champion while a student at Bryn Mawr. She was a member of the U.S. National Team from 1992 to 1995. As a coach she led Mesa College to the California Collegiate Championship in 2000. She is currently the president of the California Community College Badminton Coaches Association.

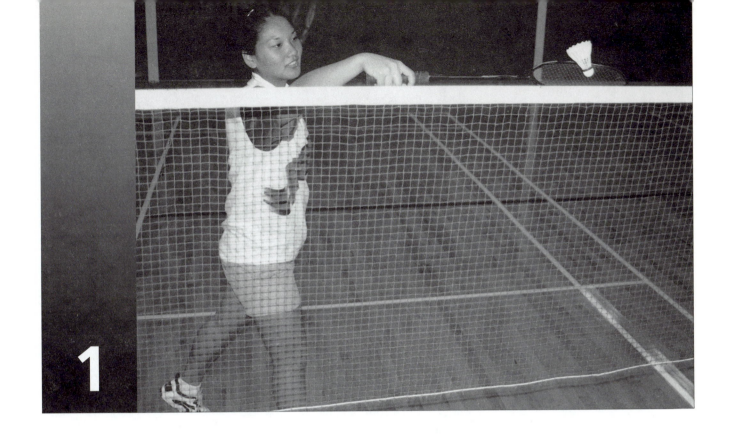

Introduction
to Badminton

Chapter Outline

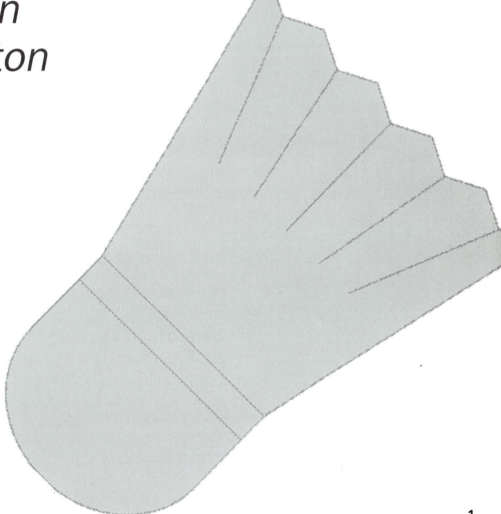

Badminton, as we know it today, is second only to soccer as the world's most popular participation activity. An activity for all ages and for both sexes, it is a unique and exciting competitive sport.

Badminton is a game in which two players (singles game) or four players (doubles game) hit a light, feathered object (shuttlecock) over a net with rackets. The objective is to win the game of 15 points (11 points for women's singles) by hitting the shuttle into the opponent's court and preventing it from landing within the boundaries of your own court. The strategy of winning involves using a variety of shots to force your opponent to lose the rally. The players attempt to move their opponents around the court, forcing weak returns, or they hit hard shots (smashes) that the opponents cannot return.

Because of the limited exposure badminton receives in the United States, many people hold the erroneous belief that it is not a vigorous and challenging activity. When observing beginners hitting the shuttle slowly over the net, it becomes easy to draw this conclusion. But given the proper instruction, the players can learn to control the tempo of the game, and it becomes fascinating to watch as well as to play. As the players learn more strokes, the rallies become more exciting.

Benefits of Playing Badminton

Badminton is one of the fastest-growing sports internationally, with over one billion people playing worldwide. It is second only to soccer as the world's most popular participation activity. Badminton can be played indoors or outdoors, by anyone at any age—it is a true lifetime sport. It is the easiest of all the racket sports to learn, and beginners are quickly able to rally. Whether played as family recreation or in tournament competition, badminton is fast and addictive.

At the advanced level, badminton is the fastest racket sport as the shuttle can travel at speeds up to 200 miles per hour. Despite the court being relatively small (20 by 44 feet), badminton will require top players to run 3 to 5 miles in a match with a one-minute rally consisting of 20 or more changes of direction.

Badminton at every level is an excellent cardiovascular activity with its long rallies. Stretching and twisting aid in developing flexibility. The fast pace of the game improves hand-eye coordination, sharpens both physical and mental reflexes, and is great exercise.

On a psychological level, badminton helps reduce tensions as players move around the court and strike the shuttle. Additionally, as they improve in skill, they develop a higher level of self-satisfaction that comes with the accomplishment of any goal.

Many racket sports are difficult and frustrating to learn. In badminton, even beginning players can start a rally almost immediately and gain a sense of achievement. Whether you are playing just for the exercise or planning to enter competition, it is an excellent cardiovascular activity. It requires fast reflexes, good physical conditioning, and concentration.

Furthermore, badminton is a lifetime sport, not just one for the young. It is fun for everyone, so grab your partner and get started!

History of Badminton

Although some evidence indicates that a game similar to badminton (called *battledore*) was played in China 2,000 years ago, badminton as it is presently played originated in England. The English royal court records refer to a similar sport as early as the 12th century. Most historians believe that English officers brought the game they called *Poona* to India in the 17th century. They then brought it back home again to England in the late 19th century. In 1873 they played Poona at the Duke of Beaufort's estate, called Badminton House, near the village of Badminton in Gloucestershire, England. The name of the duke's estate soon became the name of the game. It was from this time that the game began to develop rapidly as a popular pastime.

The first badminton club was formed in Bath, England, in 1873. The game was introduced to North America in the 1890s. In 1895 the National Badminton Association of America was formed, and in 1899 the first All England championship tournament for men was played. The next year the championship for women was inaugurated.

As the sport gained in popularity, it became necessary to establish the rules, equipment, and court dimensions. Eventually, in 1893 the English Badminton Association was organized to bring some uniformity in competition.

The rules, called *laws,* have changed little since this time.

In 1909, the shuttle that we use today was introduced. Prior to this time very fast and unpredictable *missiles* made with poultry feathers arbitrarily stuck into a piece of cork were used. The court was originally shaped like a wasp or hourglass. Today the court is rectangular, and the tournament shuttles are made of very uniform goose feathers inserted into a precisely shaped cork base. In earlier days, the racket was heavy, but modern technology has produced a dramatic change in weight.

Since 1929, badminton has increased in popularity in the United States. The game is played in clubs and in competition between high schools and colleges across the country.

It has been a full Olympic medal sport since 1992 with China, Denmark, Indonesia, Korea, and Malaysia dominating international competition in men's singles, women's singles, men's doubles, women's doubles, and mixed doubles.

Many local and national tournaments and a world championship for individuals are held regularly. In addition, national teams compete for the Thomas Cup (similar to the Davis Cup in tennis) for men and the Uber Cup for women. Three singles matches and two doubles matches decide the winner in each competition.

Where to Play Badminton

Many high schools and colleges have badminton classes and recreation opportunities. Public parks and recreation centers also often offer opportunities to play, as do many YMCAs and YWCAs. Private badminton clubs are located in most parts of the United States. For more specific information, contact the United States Badminton Association, 501 W. Sixth Street, Papillion, Nebraska 68046 (phone: 402-592-7309).

Summary

1. Badminton as we know it originated in England.

2. It is a sport that can be enjoyed at any age—a lifetime sport.

3. Badminton can be as slow and relaxing or as vigorous and taxing as you want it to be.

4. The game requires speed, finesse, cardiovascular endurance, and strength.

Checklist on the Basics of the Game

1. Most games are completed with 15 points. Women's singles games end at 11 points.

2. Only the server can score.

3. During a rally the players attempt to get their opponents to miss a shot by forcing them out of position or hitting a hard shot that cannot be returned.

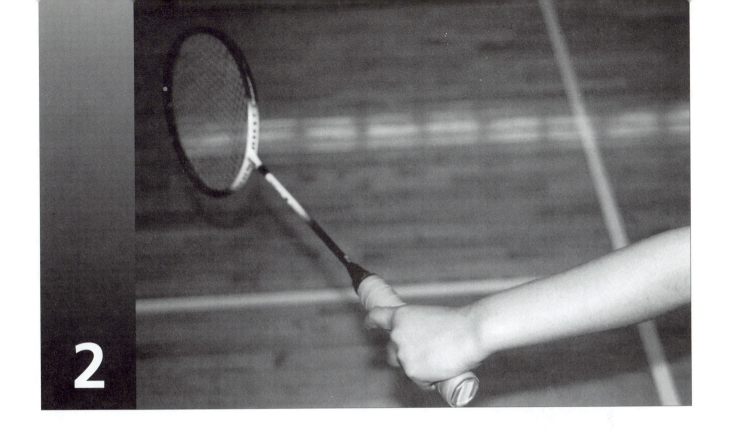

2

Equipment and Facilities

Chapter Outline

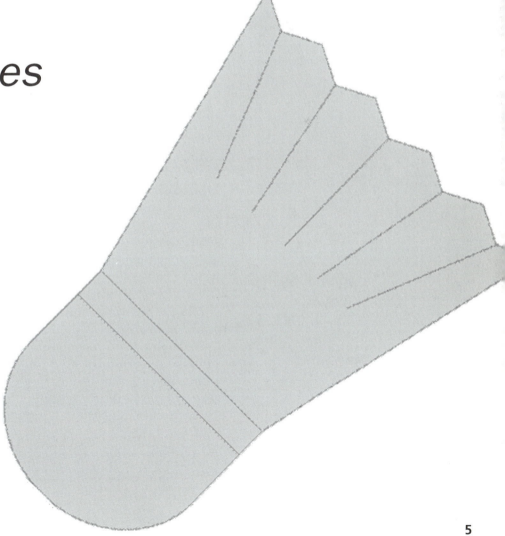

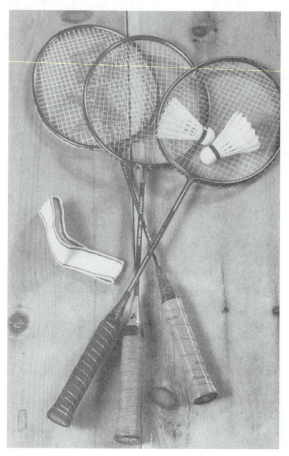

Rackets

The Racket

Badminton rackets are very light due to the quick nature of the game. Most rackets today weigh between 80 and 100 grams and are made of high-modulus graphite, titanium, carbon, graphite-fiberglass composite, aluminum, or steel. Rackets range in prices from $10 to $170.

Beginning players should start with a metal racket as their construction will allow them to make mistakes while learning to play. More advanced players should select a one-piece racket that is appropriate for their style of play.

If you enter into competitive badminton, you will soon decide whether to be primarily an offensive or a defensive player. An offensive player hits hard and tries to score points by attacking and is hunting for the winner from midcourt or the net. A defensive player tries to return every shot back and waits for the opponent to make the mistake by playing an all-court game. Every player must have both offensive and defensive skills, but most players will emphasize one style or the other.

Offensive-minded players generally use stiffer rackets that are more heavily weighted on the head. This gives the player more potential power in a shot. Defensive players use light-headed rackets.

The *head,* or *face,* of the racket is strung with synthetic strings. Natural gut is rarely used in badminton today. Nylon shuttle users require more durable strings due to the weight of the shuttle on the string bed. Players can select from a variety of synthetic strings to fit their playing needs.

The grip is the part of the handle covered with leather or polyurethane. Badminton grips are usually small—the range in circumference is from 3⅛ to 3½ inches. Overgrips and towel grips are useful to build up the grip to increase comfort and to prevent racket slippage.

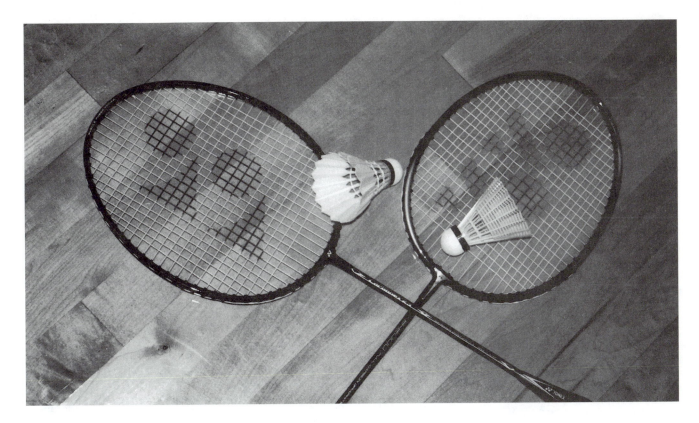

Shuttles: feather and plastic

The Shuttlecock

The *shuttlecock*, usually called the *shuttle* or *bird*, weighs about one-sixth of an ounce (more technically about 4 grams or 73 to 85 grains). The official shuttles are made of goose feathers placed in a leather-covered cork head. This is the type of shuttle used in all high-level play. Beginners and school classes often use a cheaper and more durable plastic or nylon shuttle.

When the temperature is high or you are playing at a higher altitude, air is thinner. You will then want a lighter shuttle so that it will fall more slowly. Heavier shuttles are used closer to sea level, in climates with a higher humidity, and for outdoor playing.

Clothing

Men and women alike usually wear shorts and shirts, although some women wear tennis dresses or skirts. The preferred color is white. It helps disguise the white shuttlecock (seen against the backdrop of white clothing)—especially when a player is serving. While most clubs and tournaments allow the same kinds of clothing worn for tennis, some specify a particular type and color. It is wise to check with the director to determine local requirements.

Shirts usually are made of cotton because it has better perspiration-absorption qualities than synthetic fabrics. All clothing should allow you to stretch comfortably.

Due to the quick starting and stopping involved, a badminton shoe is preferred. It should have a nonmarking sole with nonskid tread and good flexibility. The shoes should be lightweight and comfortable and provide lateral foot stability.

Badminton shoes should be low cut to allow the Achilles heel tendon to stretch while lunging and recovering. Do not use tennis shoes, running shoes, basketball shoes, or shoes designed for other sports.

The socks should be white and made of wool or cotton to absorb perspiration. To avoid blisters, you may want to wear two pairs of lighter socks. The two socks rub against each other and reduce the friction between the shoe and the skin that might otherwise result in a blister.

If you perspire heavily, you might want to wear a sweatband on your forehead. The sweatband reduces the perspiration that can run into your eyes and also keeps your hair away from your face. Wristbands prevent perspiration from rolling down your arm and getting your hand sweaty, possibly causing your grip to slip.

The Court

The badminton court is 44 feet long. The singles court is 17 feet wide, and the doubles court is 20 feet wide. The lines are inbounds. The top of the net is 5 feet, 1 inch, at the post and 5 feet at the center of the court.

There is a short service line 6 feet, 6 inches, from the net. The server must stand behind this line, in the service court area, and the serve must clear the opposite short service line to be in play.

The serving court for singles is bounded by the short service line, the centerline, the singles sideline, and the back boundary of the court. This produces a long, narrow court of 15 feet, 6 inches long and 8 feet, 6 inches wide. The server must stand within this court and serve into the diagonally opposite singles court to have a legal serve.

The doubles service court is shorter but wider than the singles court. It is bounded by the short service line in front, the centerline, the doubles sideline and a line 2 feet, 6 inches in from the rear boundary. The doubles server must stand in this court and serve to the diagonally opposite doubles court to begin play.

There should be at least 20 feet of clearance overhead—24 to 30 feet is considered ideal. A 30-foot ceiling is required for national and international competition.

Court: Top view

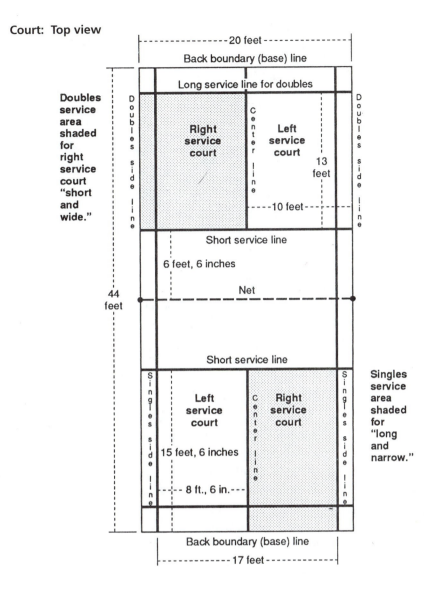

Doubles service area shaded for right service court "short and wide."

20 feet

Back boundary (base) line

Long service line for doubles

Doubles side line

Right service court

Center line

Left service court

13 feet

10 feet

Doubles side line

Short service line

6 feet, 6 inches

Net

44 feet

Short service line

Singles side line

Left service court

Center line

Right service court

Singles side line

15 feet, 6 inches

8 ft., 6 in.

Singles service area shaded for "long and narrow."

Back boundary (base) line

17 feet

Court: Side view

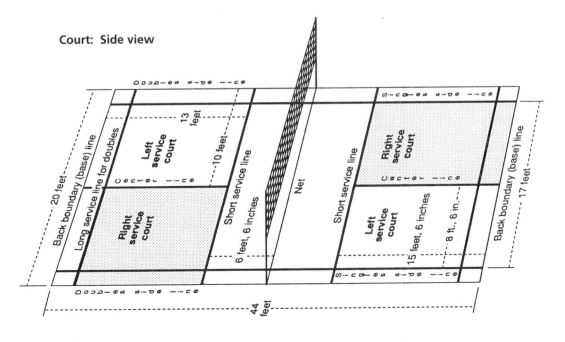

Checklist for Game or Practice Equipment

1. One or two rackets
2. Two tubes of shuttlecocks
3. Shirt and shorts
4. Shoes and socks
5. Towel
6. Sweatbands for forehead and wrist (optional)

Summary

1. Rackets can be made of wood, metal, or other materials.

2. Offensive players generally use a racket heavier in the head than the racket defensive players would choose.

3. The shuttlecock can be made of feathers and cork or nylon. The plastic or nylon shuttle plays longer, but the feathers give a better flight and a steeper drop.

4. Clothing should be comfortable enough to allow you to run unimpaired and to stretch easily. The preferred color is white.

5. Badminton shoes have flexible and nonskid soles.

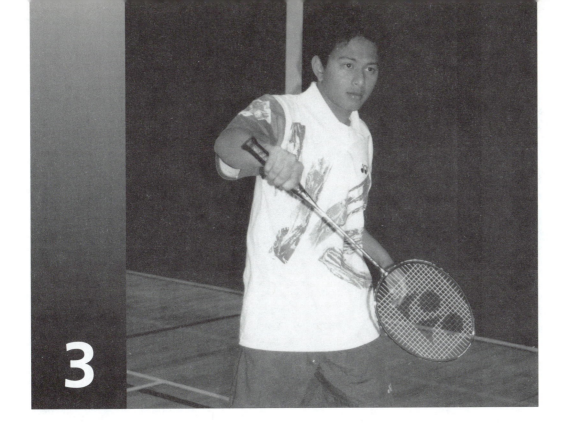

3

Getting Started

Chapter Outline

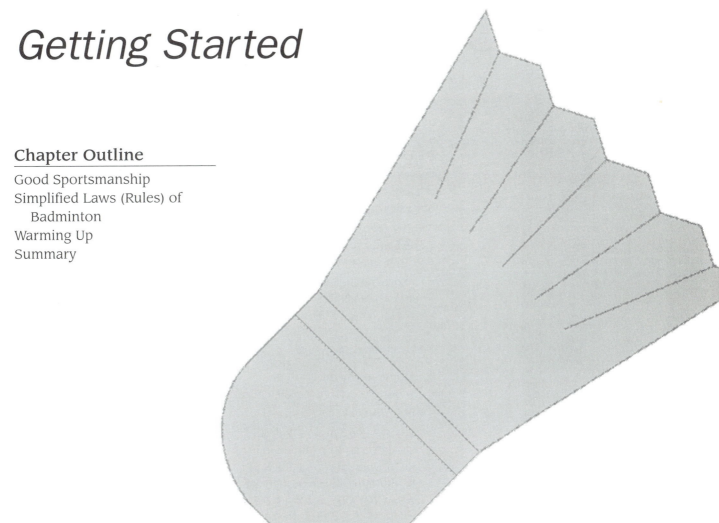

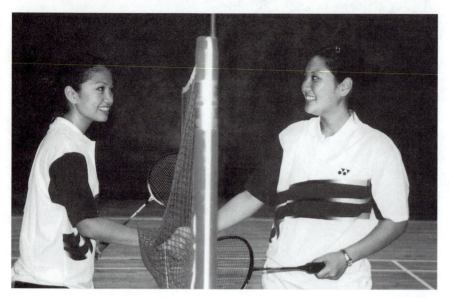

Opponents shaking hands

Good Sportsmanship

The game of badminton emphasizes good sportsmanship, expressed through certain playing *courtesies*. It is expected that you will be friendly to and respectful of your opponent and gracious whether winning or losing. In addition, here are some specific courtesies expected from those who play badminton:

1. Introduce yourself to your partner and to your opponents before the match. Be sure to shake hands after the match.

2. While warming up, help your opponent's warm-up as well; don't kill every stroke.

3. If there is any question on whether you have fouled, call it on yourself.

4. When you are in doubt about whether a shuttle landed in or out, always give the benefit of the doubt to your opponent or replay the point.

5. Never question your opponent's calls.

6. While at times during a match you may want to aim a smash at your opponent, do not do it if you can get the point any other way. If you have a setup, hit it somewhere else in the court.

7. Control your anger. Never throw your racket.

8. Never deride or make fun of an opponent.

9. As the server, keep the score and call it before each serve, calling the server's score first.

10. When your opponent is serving and a shuttle lands out of bounds on your side of the court, pick it up and hit it back, or toss it under the net to the server.

11. Compliment your opponent on any good shots made.

12. Do not offer advice or criticism to your partner or your opponents.

13. Bring your share of shuttlecocks to every practice and game.

14. Keep up the play. Do not stall between points.

15. Do not talk to your partner during a rally except when you are directing tactics, as in "I've got it" or "You're up."

16. If you are receiving, be ready to return the shuttle as soon as the server is ready to serve.

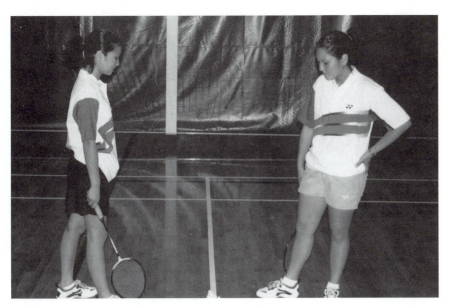

Deciding who serves first by a toss of the shuttle

Simplified Laws (Rules) of Badminton

The complete laws of the game will be found in the appendix of this book. A summary follows:

1. Toss for the serve. You can flip a coin, spin a racket, or toss a shuttle to determine who gets the choice of "side or serve." If spinning a racket, identify a marking on the racket and then spin it in the hand or on the floor. One person calls the mark. If it is called correctly, that person gets the choice. The most common method of determining the choice, however, is by hitting or tossing the shuttle into the air and letting it land. The person toward whom the base of the shuttle is pointing gets the choice. If the winner of the toss chooses a side of the court to defend, the other person can choose serve or receive.

The side of the court may become important if one side has poorer lighting or an undesirable background. In an important match the player who wins the toss might elect to defend the less desirable first. This would then have him or her on the best side for the last half of the third game.

2. For women's singles, games are played to 11 points. All other singles and doubles games are played to 15 points.

In a 15-point game, if the score is tied at 14–14, the player who scored 14 first can decide to play one more point (no set) or three more points (set) to finish the game. In an 11-point game, if the game is tied at 10–10, the player who scored 10 first has choice between one and three more points.

Once the score is set, the player who tied the score continues to serve.

3. The serve, if not played by the receiver, must land in the diagonal service court. Any shuttle hitting the line is *in*. In singles the shuttle must land in the long, narrow court. In doubles it must land in the short, wide court. In doubles the long service line is for the service boundary only. Once the serve has been hit, the full court (20 by 44 feet) is played.

In singles the serve is made from the right service court whenever the server's score is an even number (0, 2, 4, etc.). The serve is from the left court whenever the server's score is an odd number (1, 3, 5, etc.).

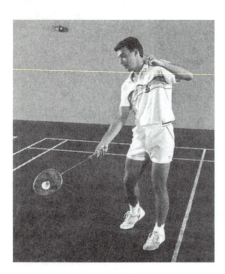

Correct serve

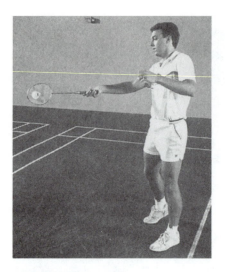

Incorrect serve:
A. Above the waist

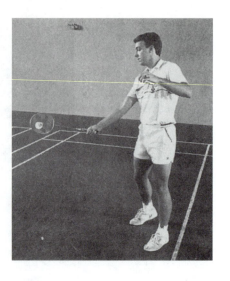

B. Racket head above the hand

In doubles the serve is always started from the right court. The first server in doubles will serve from the right court. If the point is won, the server will serve next from the left court. The server will alternate sides until the serve is lost. The players on both teams should remember where they were during the first service, because they will have to be in those same positions whenever the server's score is even. The returners will always defend the same service court during an *inning*—that is, the time that a player or team holds service. (Once the serve has been returned, the players can move anyplace in the court.) The servers will change courts whenever they score.

In doubles the first server serves until the serving team commits a fault, and the serve is lost. This is called *one hand down*. When the first serving team loses the serve, the opponent in the right court (the receiver in the first hand) will

serve and will continue to serve until the serve is lost. Then the server's partner will serve until the serve is lost. Then the server's partner will serve until the serve is lost—*two hands down*. The players on the team that began serving in the match will then each get a turn and serve until losing.

4. The server has only one chance to serve the shuttle over the net and into the proper court. The shuttle may hit the net and land in the proper court and be legal.

5. Most matches are best two out of three games. The winner of the match will be the one who wins two games. The players will change sides of the court after each game. If a third game is required, the players will switch ends after 8 points in a 15-point game and after 6 points in an 11-point game.

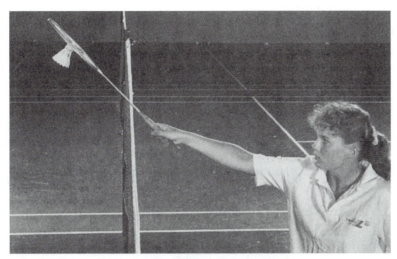

Reaching over the net to return the shuttle

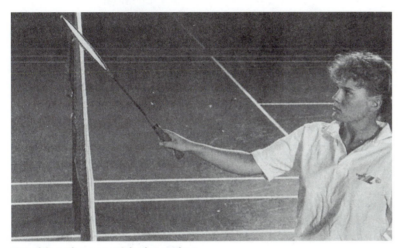

Touching the net with the racket

6. Faults (loss of serve for the serving team or loss of the point for the receiving team) occur for the following reasons:

   a. A serve is illegal because
      - the shuttle is hit when it is above the waist,
      - the head of the racket is above the hand when the shuttle is hit, or
      - the server misses the shuttle when trying to hit it.

   b. Any serve or other shot that goes under or through the net.

   c. A serve lands outside the proper service area.

   d. A shot lands out of bounds (only if the shuttle's head, not the feathers, lands outside the lines).

   e. Either the server or the receiver steps out of the proper court before the shuttle is served.

   f. The receiving player does not play the shuttle. (Only the proper receiver may return the serve.)

   g. A player reaches over the net to hit the shuttle. (It is legal to follow through over the net provided that the player or racket does not hit the net.)

   h. A player touches the net with the racket or any part of the body or clothing.

   i. A player hits the shuttle twice (a double hit) or carries it on the racket (rather than having it bounce quickly from the strings) before it crosses the net.

   j. The server steps forward when serving.

   k. A player obstructs or hinders an opponent.

   l. A player catches the shuttle and calls it *out*.

Warming Up

While traditionally it has been common to stretch prior to physical activity, research indicates that stretching before the workout is not always recommended. In fact, it may increase the risk of injury and may reduce one's potential strength. (See, e.g., G. W. Gleim and M. P. McHugh, "Flexibility and Its Effects on Sports Injury and Performance," *Sports Medicine* [New Zealand] 24, no. 5 [November 1997]: 289–299.)

A 1983 survey of 500 runners found that those who warmed up had more injuries than those who did not (87.7 percent vs. 66 percent), and the frequency of injuries increased with the length of the warm-up. It is assumed that stretching was part of the warm-up but it was not specifically asked. (See J. A. Kerner and J. C. D'Amico, "A Statistical Analysis of a Group of Runners," *Journal of the American Podiatry Association* 73, no. 3 [1983]: 160–164.) A few years later, a survey of 10K runners in the national championships found that those who stretched had more injuries. But it is not known whether those who stretched did so because they already had an injury and assumed that the stretching would protect them from further injury. (See S. J. Jacobs and B. L. Berson, "Injuries to Runners: A Study of Entrants to a 10,000 Meter Race," *American Journal of Sports Medicine* 14, no. 2 [1986]: pp. 151–155.)

One thing we know is that we are all individuals with unique potentials or problems relative to our muscles and connective tissues. Some people like to do stretching exercises as part of their warm-up; some do not. Some it may help, but some it may hurt. (For a more complete summary of the research, see B. O'Connor, *Scientific Conditioning for Female Athletes* [Terre Haute, IN: WISH, 2001].)

The research indicates that the warm-up should allow for the muscles used in the activity to warm up. So for badminton, rallying slowly, serving, and hitting overheads should suffice for the warm-up.

Summary

1. Badminton is a game in which good sportsmanship is expected.

2. The courtesies spell out the expected behavior of a badminton player.

3. The laws of badminton allow for 11-point games (for women's singles) and 15-point games (for men's singles and all doubles games).

4. When the game is tied at 1 point away from the expected game-ending score, the player or team who reached that score first may either set to three points or opt for "no set" (i.e., one point).

5. The shuttle cannot be double-hit.

6. The lines are in.

7. Players should warm up before a game or a hard practice session.

Checklist for Serving Faults

1. When serving, the shuttle must be hit with the entire racket head below the waist.

2. The head of the racket must be below the hand when the shuttle is hit.

3. The shuttle must not hit anyone before the receiver has the opportunity of hitting it. (The shuttle may hit the net.)

4. The server must have both feet in contact with the floor when beginning the serve.

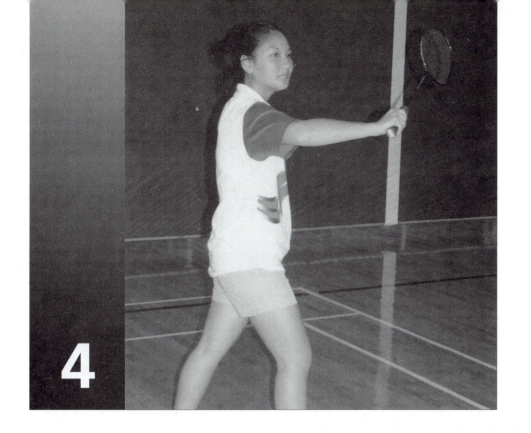

Grips, the Ready Position, and Footwork

Forehand grip:

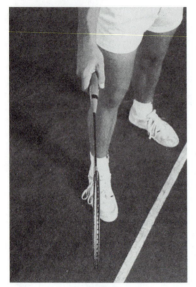

A. From above: right

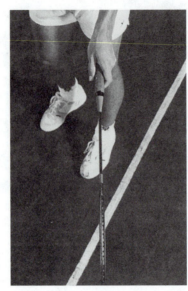

B. From above: left

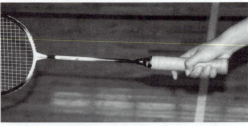

C. From side: right

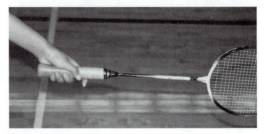

D. From side: left

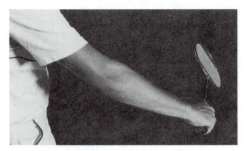

E. From back: right

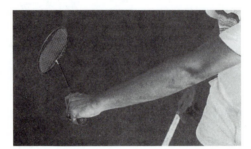

F. From back: left

Grips

The basics of badminton skills start with the grip. Without the proper grip, you will not be able to execute strokes effectively or efficiently. There are two essential grips: the forehand and the backhand. The following description is for right-handed players. If you are left-handed, just reverse the instructions. Whichever grip you use, you should check it often to make sure it is correct.

Forehand Grip

Hold the head of your racket perpendicular to the floor and "shake hands" with the grip on the handle of the racket. The juncture of your thumb and index finger will form a V, slightly left of center on the top of the grip. The grip should be with your fingers, not the palm of your hand. Your fingers should be slightly spread, with your forefinger extended higher on the handle.

Your thumb wraps around the handle and rests on the side of the middle finger. The palm of the hand should be parallel with the face of the racket. The butt of the racket handle should be touching the heel of your hand.

The grip should be loose enough so that the crook of both the middle and ring fingers have a slight gap from the handle. Gripping the racket tightly as you would a hammer will cause the muscles in your hand and forearm to be stiff. This "hammer grip" results in a loss of control.

As you hit a shot, you will squeeze the racket handle with pressure from the wrapped thumb, the index finger, and the pinky finger. When you hit with power, you will tighten your grip at these three points more than on softer shots.

Backhand Grip

For strokes taken on the backhand (nonracket) side of the body, the grip must be changed to a backhand grip. Otherwise, the racket face will point slightly upward, and you will not have control of the shot.

There are two types of backhand grips. The first has the racket moved a quarter-turn clockwise (so that as your thumb moves farther behind the racket, the back of your hand moves toward the handle). The knuckle of your index finger will now be on the top of the handle, and your thumb will be behind the handle, pointing up the shaft. The **V** formed at the base of your thumb and index finger will now be over the top bevel of the handle.

Some players believe that they have more power with this technique. The disadvantage is for shots behind you, in which the grip loses some of its effectiveness. This is also the grip used in the backhand serve.

The second type of backhand grip changes only the position of the thumb from the forehand grip. It moves from behind the handle

Checklist for the Forehand Grip

1. With the racket head perpendicular to the floor, is the V formed by the thumb and index finger on top of the handle grip?
2. Is the index finger separated from the middle finger by resting higher on the handle?
3. Is the grip loose rather than tight?
4. Is the racket held in the fingers rather than in the palm of your hand?

Checklist for the Backhand Grip

1. Did you move your hand a quarter-turn toward the back side of the handle?
2. Is the first knuckle of the index finger on top of the handle?
3. Is your thumb behind the handle and pointing up the shaft?

Backhand grip:

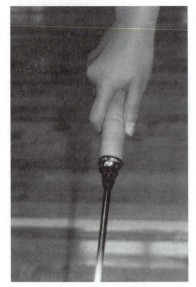

A. From above: right

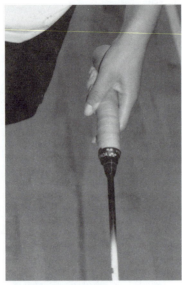

B. From above: left

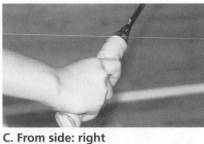

C. From side: right

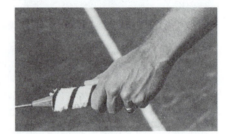

D. From side: left

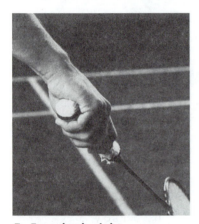

E. From back: right

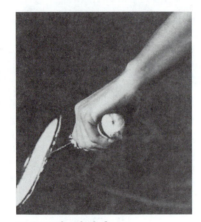

F. From back: left

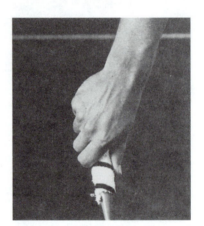

**G. Backhand grip changing
thumb position**

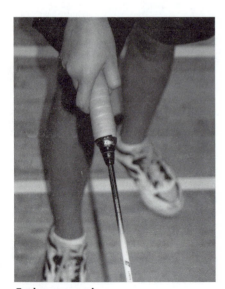

Frying-pan grip

to a position along the upper left corner of it. This grip is more efficient for shots behind you. Some players prefer it for other shots as well.

Frying-Pan Grip

Sometimes used by more advanced players, the so-called frying-pan grip is used primarily in doubles play at the net and for service returns. To get the feel of this grip, place the racket on the floor and grasp it like a frying pan about an inch above the end of the handle. This is also known as the Western grip.

Ready position for return

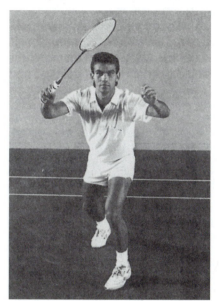

Rally-ready position

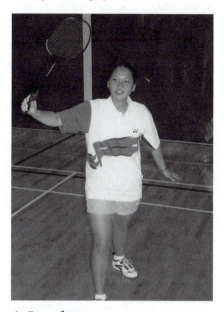

A. From front

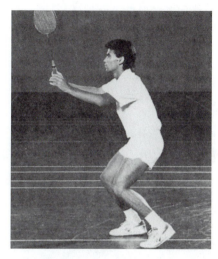

B. From side

The Ready Position

Ready position in badminton is similar to that used in many other sports. It should allow the player to move quickly in any direction. Badminton has two types of ready positions: rally ready and ready position for return of service.

Rally Ready

The rally-ready position is taken whenever you are ready to hit a shot, whether it be a smash, a drive, or a drop. From this position you will be best able to move effectively forward or back and right or left. It is similar to the ready position for most sports. Your feet should be spread to shoulder width or slightly wider. Your ankles and knees should be slightly flexed, and you should be bent forward at the waist. Your weight should be slightly on the balls of your feet so that you are ready to move in any direction. (If you curl your toes down just a bit,

you will feel your weight on the forward part of your feet.)

Your arms should be forward of your body, with the racket up and held above the hand, which is at waist-height—ready to intercept either a forehand or backhand shot. You should be well balanced and relaxed, because you can move more quickly when you are relaxed than when you are tense.

The first reaction from ready position just before your opponent hits the shuttle is to "load" both legs with the anticipation of pushing off the floor and in the direction of the shuttle.

Ready Position for Return of Service

This position is slightly different. You will keep your nonracket foot (left foot for right-handers) forward. This will allow you to move more quickly up and back as necessary to return a service. The racket head will be in front of your right shoulder for right-handers or the left shoulder for left-handers.

If the serve is behind you, push off your left foot, and run

Home base: singles

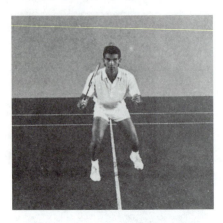

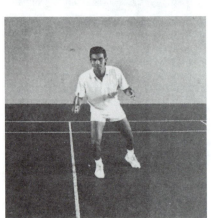

Checklist for the Ready Position

1. Are you in the center of the court?
2. Are your shoulders square to the net?
3. Are your feet spread slightly wider than your shoulders with your weight on the balls of your feet?
4. Are your ankles, knees, and hips slightly flexed so that you are ready to move in any direction?
5. Are you holding the racket with a forehand grip and with the racket forward of the midline of your body?
6. Are you ready to move in any direction quickly?

or shuffle back to the spot where you will hit the shuttle. If the serve is hit short, bring your right foot forward and attack the shuttle.

Home Base for Singles Games

In badminton you do not have time to get ready for most shots as you do in tennis or golf. For this reason, you must always be ready to react to the shuttle. The best position from which to defend your court is in the middle of the court—on the centerline, a few feet ahead of a spot halfway between the net and the back boundary line. (This puts you about 2 feet behind the T that is formed by the centerline meeting the front service line.) From this position you can get to the front court to handle the drop shots and will still have time to move back to play the clears.

Depending on your individual strength and quickness, you might want to play a few feet ahead or behind this center area. Your

home-base position may also vary depending on your opponent. You might play farther forward if the opponent is weaker or uses a lot of drop shots. You might play farther back against a strong smasher or clearing player.

As you become more advanced, you may move a bit to one side or the other to take away your opponent's angle of return. When you hit a deep corner, your opponent has a greater angle in which to return to your court. If you hit to the center of the court, the angle is reduced.

Always try to get to home base after every shot. However, if your opponent is ready to hit the shuttle and you haven't yet returned to your home base, stop and get set to defend your court from wherever you are on the court.

Footwork

Good, smooth footwork is essential to badminton. You must be able to get into position quickly

**Center position for
shot down middle**

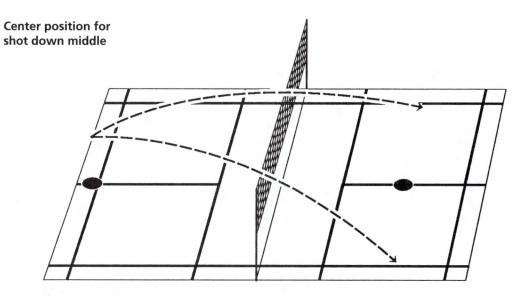

**Angle of return:
A. With opponent in
deep right corner**

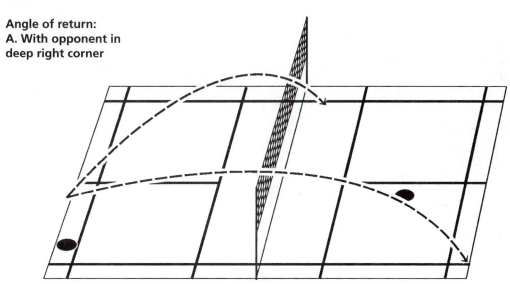

**B. With opponent in
deep left corner**

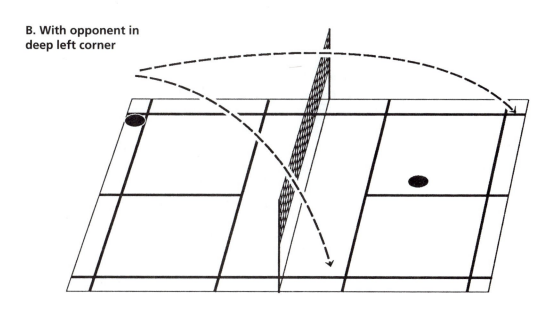

Footwork:

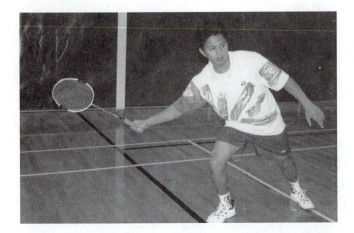

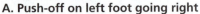

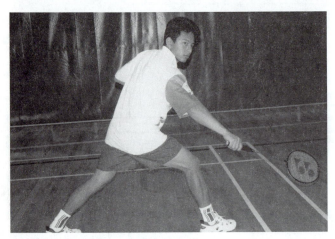

A. Push-off on left foot going right

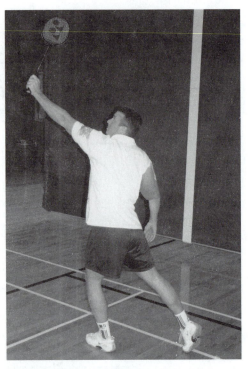

B. Turn sideways on deep shots

to hit the shuttle before you can hit your stroke. *Racket foot* in this discussion refers to right foot for right-handers.

Starting from home base, the entire court can be covered in three steps: racket foot, nonracket foot, and racket foot. Basic footwork consists of pushing off the floor using both feet, watching the shuttle as it leaves from your opponent's racket, pivoting the body, and moving on balance with the final step on the racket foot.

Movement on the court must be fluid, rhythmic, and efficient. As leg strength improves and stride increases, you can reduce the number of steps required to cover areas of the court to two steps: step with nonracket foot and lunge with the racket foot. If the shuttle is close or there is little time to react, just stretch with the racket foot.

The grace and ease with which top-level badminton players move to all the corners of the badminton court require great agility, speed, strength, and endurance. Quick and light footwork comes from repetitive and physically demanding practice of on-court movement. Shuttle runs (without

Step with racket foot toward net on shots hit close to the net:

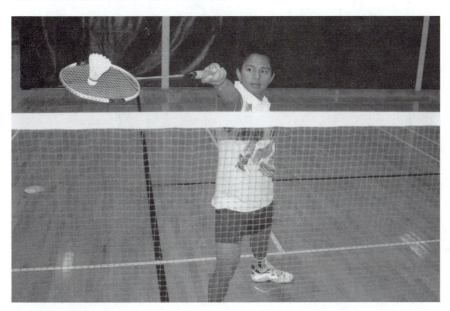

A. Right court

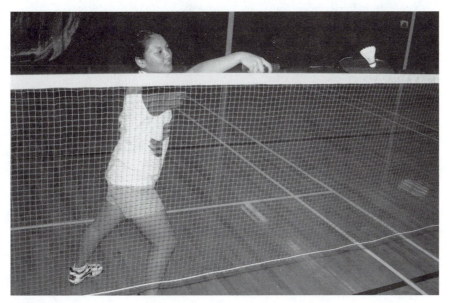

B. Left court

racket) and shadow practice (with racket) are two standard methods of improving footwork:

Shuttle runs: Set up three to five shuttles (cork end up) in the forehand forecourt. Starting from home base, move to forehand net, lunge on racket foot and pick up first shuttle, return to home base, continue to move to backhand net, and place the shuttle (cork up) on the ground. Return to home base and repeat until all five shuttles moved from forehand net to backhand net.

With six corners of the court—forehand and backhand forecourt, forehand and backhand midcourt, and forehand and backhand backcourt—proficiency in court movement will require being able to make the transition to all 15 combinations of the six corners. As movement skills progress, increase the number of shuttles and the number of combinations practiced per session.

Shadow practice: Your partner stands at the net and points to the various corners where he or she has "hit" an imaginary shuttle. Visualize responding to your opponent's shot, move quickly to that corner, and swing your racket as if you were hitting your response. Quickly return to the home base, in the center of the court, after each shot. Switch with your partner when the quality of movements declines or after a set number of movements.

Scissors step on smash

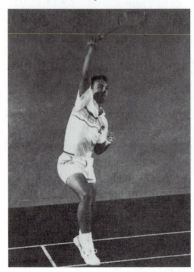 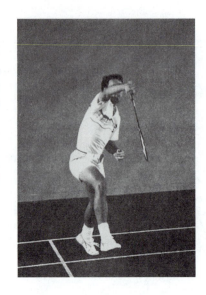 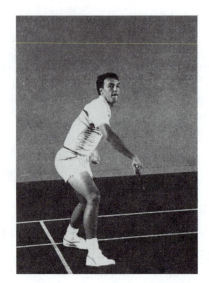

Summary

1. The grip is very important. Without the proper grip for the chosen stroke, you will drastically reduce your chances of making an effective shot.

2. The ready position is similar to that used in many other sports. It should allow the player to move quickly in any direction.

3. Always have your racket up and ready so that you can take the offense.

4. The home-base position is in midcourt and slightly forward of the midpoint of the centerline.

5. Good footwork is essential in badminton.

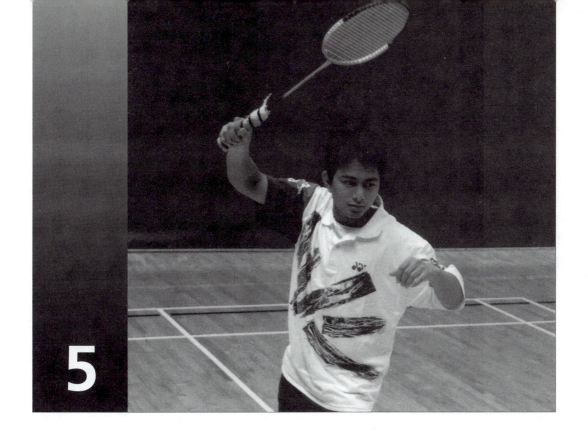

Service
and Service Return

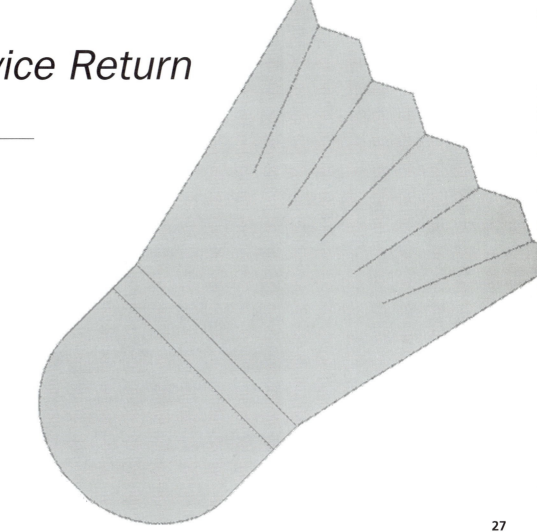

High deep serve:

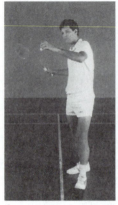

A.

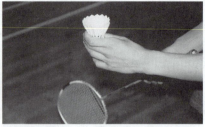

B.

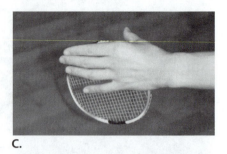

C.

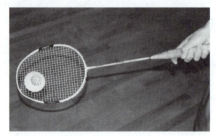

D.

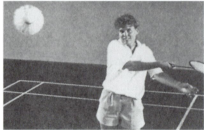

E.

A. Two to three feet from T
B. Fingers gripping shuttle at base, racket ready
C. Drop shuttle
D. Contact (right)
E. Contact (left)
F. Follow-through

F.

The Serve

The serve should be learned first, since all rallies start with one. Also, it is through the serve that a player begins to "control the point."

The rules state that, when serving, you must stand in the service court, and your feet must both stay in contact with the floor until after the shuttle is hit. During your arm action, your racket must contact the shuttle below your waist, and the entire head of your racket must be below your hand.

High, Deep Serve

The high, deep service is used primarily in singles play. If not hit by your opponent, this serve should land as close as possible to his or her back line. The objective is to move your opponent deep into the backcourt.

Take a position approximately 2 to 3 feet from the front service line and close to the centerline. (The point where the centerline meets the front service line is often called the *T*.) Stand with your feet comfortably apart (about shoulder width), with your racket-side foot back (the right foot for right-handed players). Your knees should be slightly bent.

Hold the shuttle by its cork base between the thumb and the index and middle finger of your left hand. Extend your left arm outward in front of the right shoulder. This allows you to hit the shuttle near waist level and in front of you. Many beginners tend to hold the shuttle low, near waist level, then drop it. This forces them to hit it at too low a point. You always want the shuttle at as high a point as is legally possible.

High, deep serve

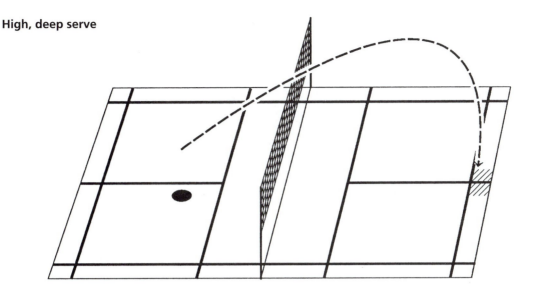

Your right wrist will be cocked up and back so that the racket head will be raised and the wrist will be at or above waist level. Your weight will be on your rear (right) foot.

As you drop the shuttle in front and to the side of your body (at about a 45-degree angle), your weight will shift forward (to your left foot), and you will swing the racket through the shuttle. At the contact point, the entire head of the racket must be below the level of your hand and below waist level.

Your body rotates in the direction of the shuttle's flight, and your wrist straightens and snaps the racket through the shuttle. You should be hitting up and out.

Follow through over your left shoulder, and let your forearm continue its rotation. Remember that you are not allowed to move or slide either foot until after contact is made with the shuttle.

The only difference in your stance between serving from the right and left courts is that when you are serving from the left, your back foot will be farther behind your front foot.

Checklist for High, Deep Serve

1. Do I have a forehand grip?
2. Is my nonracket hand extended outward to where the shuttle can be dropped effectively?
3. Is my racket behind my body with the wrist cocked?
4. Did I drop the shuttle before I started the racket forward?
5. Was the shuttle dropped to the racket side of my body?
6. Did I contact the shuttle at about knee height?
7. Did I bring the racket through quickly by using the power of my wrist and forearm?
8. Did I follow through over my nonracket shoulder?
9. Did I hit the shuttle up and out?

The most common error for beginners is bringing the racket forward before dropping the shuttle. This results in missing it completely—a fault.

Since the shuttlecock is very light and designed to catch a great deal of air in its flight, it drops slowly. Your racket swing must compensate for this slow drop. So the idea is to drop the shuttle and then hit it after it is already dropping.

Low, Short Serve

The low, short serve is used more often in doubles than in singles. The doubles service court is not as long as the singles service court, so the high, clear serves cannot be hit deeply. But since the doubles service court is wider than the singles court, the short serves can be placed farther from the receiver. In addition, the low serve forces your opponent to hit the shuttle up and gives you the opportunity to take the offensive by hitting the shuttle down.

It takes a great deal of practice to be able to serve the shuttle low over the net and to land it close to the front corners of your opponent's service court. When used in singles, this serve can keep your opponent off balance or bring him or her closer to the net so that the deep serves will be more effective.

Take a position about 2 to 3 feet from the front service line and close to the centerline. Both arms will stay close to your body while your weight rests on your forward foot.

Drop the shuttle before you start your racket forward. Your wrist will be cocked backward and upward. It will stay cocked throughout the stroke—even during the follow-through. Drop the shuttle in front of, and to the side of, your body, and swing the racket in a nearly horizontal plane around your body—with the racket head just below waist level. The racket head should be angled slightly upward to direct the shuttle just over the net. Gently guide the shuttle forward so that it just clears the net. Beginners should clear the net by 12 inches or less, advanced players by no more than 2 inches. The serve should then fall into your opponent's service area just past the service line. If the shuttle touches the net but still falls into the correct service court, it is a legal serve. The short serves should fall just past the service line. Try to hit either of the front corners of the opponent's service court. The short serve requires a great deal of practice.

Checklist for the Low, Short Serve

1. Do I have a forehand grip?
2. Is most of my weight on my forward foot?
3. Are my elbows bent and close to my waist?
4. Is my right hand near my right hip?
5. Is my wrist cocked backward?
6. Did I drop the shuttle before I started my racket swing?
7. Was the shuttle dropped to the front and right side of my body?
8. At contact did my wrist remain cocked?
9. Did I guide the shuttle over the net with my right forearm?

Short service drop:

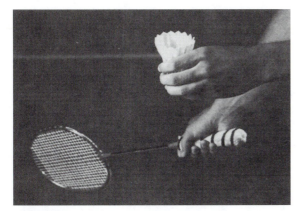

A. Ready

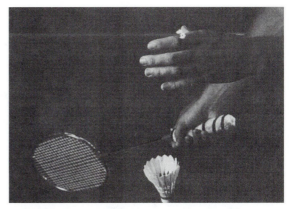

B. Drop

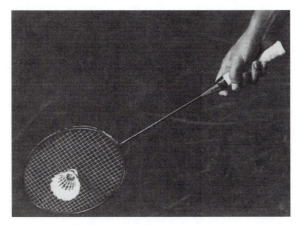

C. Contact (right)

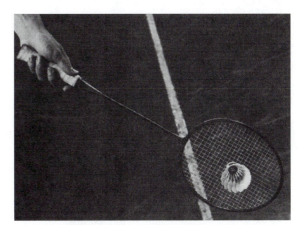

D. Contact (left)

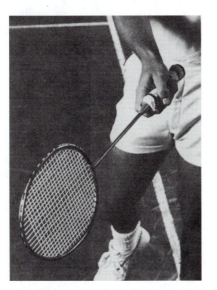

E. Follow-through (right)

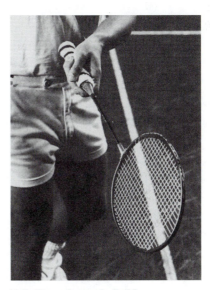

F. Follow-through (left)

Low, short serve

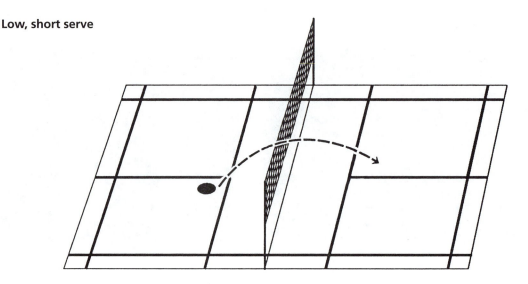

Flick Serve

The flick serve is a harder-hit serve with a low trajectory, just high enough to clear the outstretched racket when your opponent is reaching up to return it. It is used in both singles and doubles— most often in doubles, when your opponent often rushes your short serve.

The shuttle is dropped in front and away from the body. The flick serve should look just like a short serve, except that as the racket nears the shuttle, its speed is accelerated to drive the shuttle to the back court by uncocking the wrist. If the serve is not returned, it should land deep in your opponent's back court.

Drive Serve

The drive serve is hit hard but lower than a flick serve. It is used more often in doubles, when your opponent is expecting a short serve. Doubles teams that play a side-by-side alignment may find it especially valuable because it can force a weak return. Beginners may occasionally use this serve in singles, but advanced players do not, because it is easy for the advanced opponent to reach and cut it off.

Backhand Serve

The backhand *serve* is used in doubles as a more effective method of serving the low, short serve. It was developed in Indonesia in the 1960s and is now becoming popular in Western countries. This serve involves very little backswing, and the shuttlecock is hit just after it leaves the hand. Consequently, it takes less time to clear the net, giving your opponent less time to adjust to your serve. Also, because the white shuttle blends in with the white clothing of the player, it is more difficult for the receiver to see.

For this serve your stance will be parallel to the net. (When your shoulders and an imaginary line touching the front of the toes on each of your feet are parallel to the net, your stance is parallel. Some players will have only their racket-side foot forward.) Your grip will be the true backhand grip, with your thumb behind the racket handle.

Thumb and index finger should lightly grip just one or two feathers of the shuttle, holding it just below your waist and parallel to the face of the racket. Some

Flick serve:

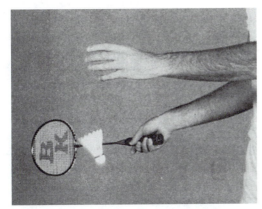

A. Drop

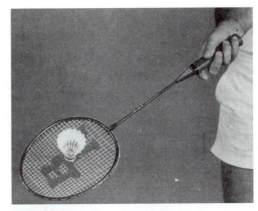

B. Contact

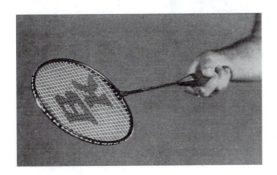

C. Follow-through

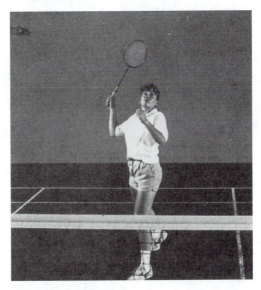

D. Speed of shuttle accelerates drive into opponent's back court

Drive serve

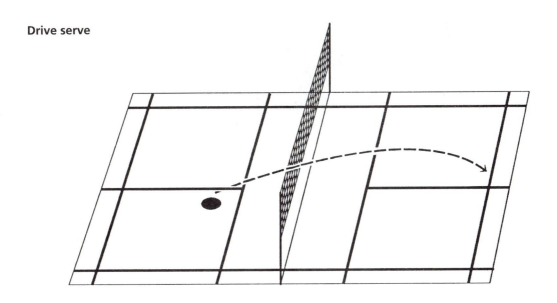

Backhand serve:

Gripping shuttle for backhand serve

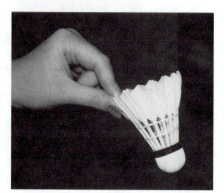

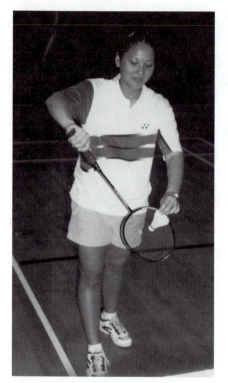

A. From front

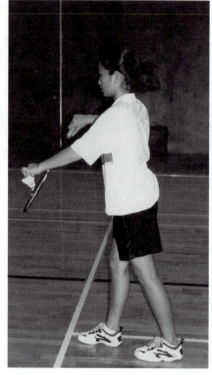

B. From side

How to hold racket for backhand serve:

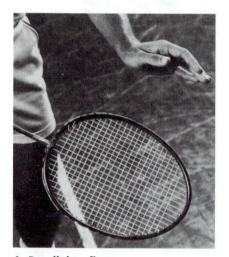

A. Parallel to floor

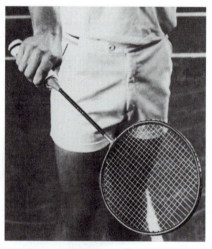

B. Perpendicular to floor

people like the racket face perpendicular to the floor; others like the face opened toward the ceiling. Whichever racket position you choose, the shuttle should be parallel to the racket face.

Your right elbow will be shoulder high, and your right arm will be away from your body. Your forearm and racket extend at a 45-degree angle downward. Remember that the shuttle has to be hit below the waist to be legal. It should just barely clear the net, landing close to your opponent's serve line.

For variation, this serve can be hit harder and become a flick or a drive serve.

> ### Checklist for Low, Backhand Serve
>
> 1. Do I have a backhand grip with the thumb behind the handle?
> 2. Is my grip higher on the handle, away from the base?
> 3. Is my stance parallel to the net?
> 4. Am I holding the shuttle below my waist and by the tip of the feathers?
> 5. Is my racket arm elbow shoulder high and away from my body?
> 6. Is the racket head angled down behind the shuttle?
> 7. Did I "push" the shuttle over the net?
> 8. Did the shuttle start dropping before it passed to the other side of the net?

Service Return

Your body position for the service return is as follows: left shoulder and foot forward; feet spread about 2 feet apart, with most of your weight on your forward foot so that you can move backward more quickly; and knees and ankles flexed, with weight on the balls of your feet. Your torso is flexed forward, and your racket is held up above your head and ready to hit.

Singles Returns

Your position on the court will be slightly forward of midcourt and slightly to the backhand side of your service court. To return a singles serve, you would be a bit deeper. From the left court, you will be the same distance back but closer to the center of the service court—the midline between the sideline and the centerline. Your alignment should allow you to protect your backhand so that you have a greater chance of playing the return with a forehand.

Watch the shuttle before it is served, and be alert for any possible serve. Then get to it as quickly as possible to catch it at its highest point. Hitting lazy underhand returns puts no pressure on the serving team.

On short serves, quickly lunge forward to the net. Your best choices of a return shot are (1) a drop to the front corner away from your opponent or (2) a high clear. On the deeper flick serves, jump back quickly, and hit a drop or a smash.

Your best strategy is to place your shot in an area of the court that forces your opponents to play defense. Use high clears to the backhand corners and drops along the net. The most effective types of returns are

- clear return,
- attacking clear return,
- smash or half-smash, and
- drop return.

The *clear return* (also used in doubles) is a high shot that clears the opponent and lands just inside the back line. Keep it away from your opponent, preferably to the backhand side. Make your opponent move. This is especially effective if you have been hitting drop returns, leading your opponent to anticipate another drop and thus come to the net. As with other clearing shots, you will

Singles service return:

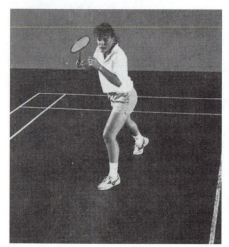

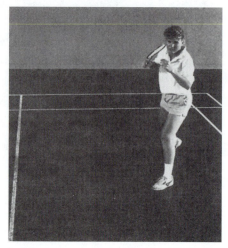

A. Right court

B. Left court

Targets for service returns

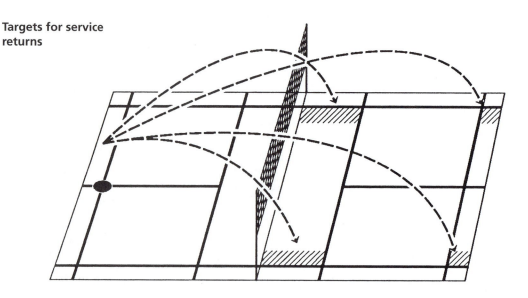

need a strong wrist action and a follow-through along the intended line of flight.

The *attacking clear return* can be used if the opponent has hit a high, weak serve and is close to the net. The trajectory in this return is lower, so the opponent has less time to react to the shot. It is aimed just like the regular clear return. The danger in this return is that if the opponent is quick to react, he or she can cut the shuttle off and smash it.

The *smash* or *half-smash* return can be used when a clear serve is too short or too low. It puts your opponent on the defensive by forcing an upward hit.

The *drop return* can be used anytime you want to move your opponent away from the center position. If your opponent has hit a drop serve, you can counter with an underhand drop return close to the net.

Two flight patterns for overhead clears

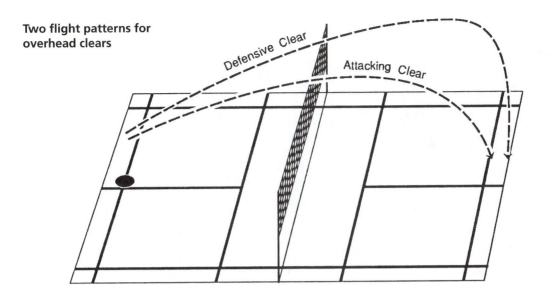

Trajectories of short clear serve and half-smash returns

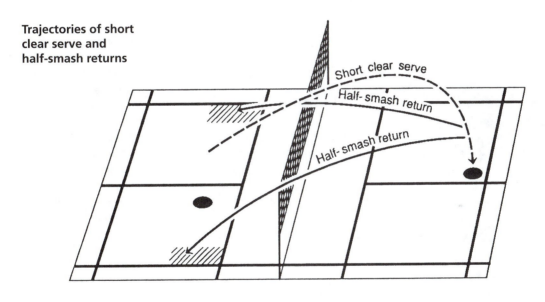

Drop return

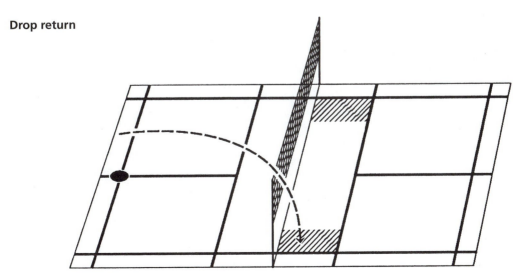

Position for doubles return

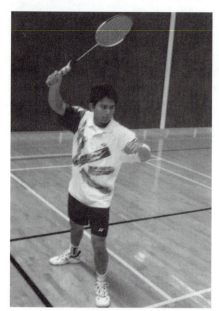

A. Right court

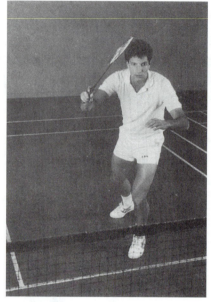

B. Left court

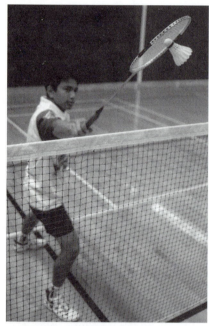

Short service return attack in doubles

Doubles Returns

Stand within a foot of the front service line and within a foot of the center service line. This will allow you to attack the low serve quickly and force your opponents to play defense.

Returns of doubles serves should be aggressive to force opponents either to clear back the shuttle or miss completely. The most effective service returns are hit sharply downward:

- Hard drive to the deep corners
- Half-court pushes to the sidelines (into the alley)
- Close drops to net

The last resort in returning doubles serve is the clear return as you start off the rally in a defensive position. Vary your returns to keep your opponents off balance.

The *hard drive return* is hit along the sidelines with a short and fast backswing. It should almost always be hit straight down the near sideline. Push off with racket leg and move racket forward with arm extended and racket head parallel to the net. At the highest point possible above the net, punch the shuttle in quick, flat motion past the server's partner.

The *half-court push return* is hit downward toward the doubles alley just behind the server but in front of the server's partner. When placed correctly, the half-court push falls low behind the net player and forces the backcourt player to hit up. It is a difficult shot because it must be played nearly perfectly or your opponents may gain the advantage.

The *doubles drop return* must be very close to the net and hit to the nearest sideline to force the server to move quickly. (Unless your opponent is out of position, do not hit the drop shot crosscourt.)

The *clear return* is the same as that used in singles.

The *doubles drive return* is hit along the sidelines with a short, fast backswing. It is used if your opponents are playing up and back and should always be hit straight down the near sideline.

Contact the shuttle in front of your body and within 2 feet of the net. It is hit flat, with the racket head parallel to the net. Only the wrist is used in this shot. If it is a backhand shot, make certain that your thumb is behind the handle in a good backhand grip.

The *push return* is a nearly sidearm return (backhand or forehand) that is pushed with the forearm into the deep backhand corner, deep forehand corner, or into your opponent's body. It starts downward from your racket.

Doubles return targets

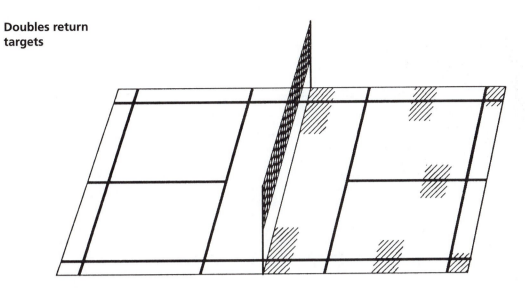

Short serve in doubles with drop return

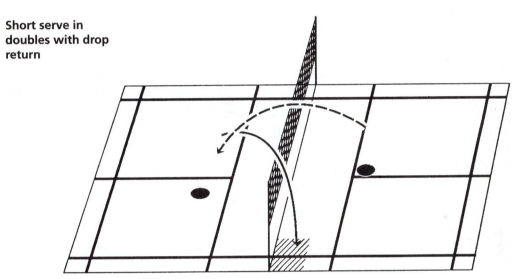

Short serve with doubles return drop

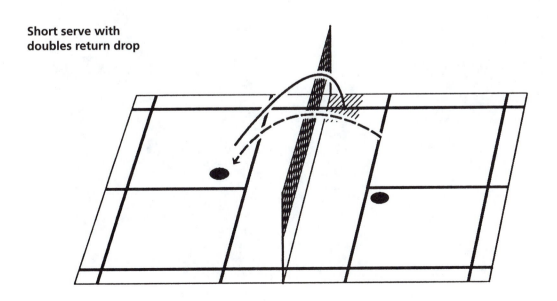

Target trajectory for half-court push return

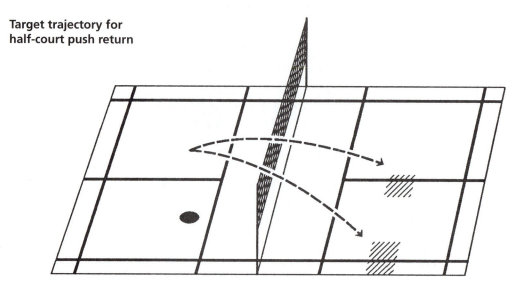

Doubles drive return

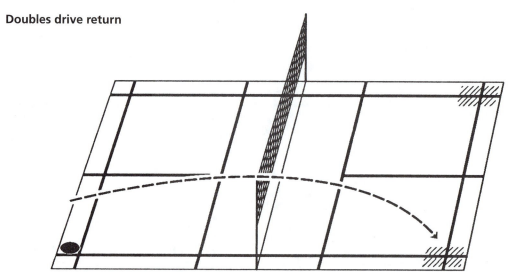

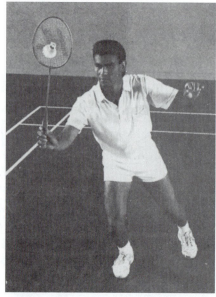

Doubles drive return contact

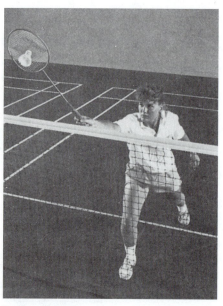

Push return contact

Push return targets

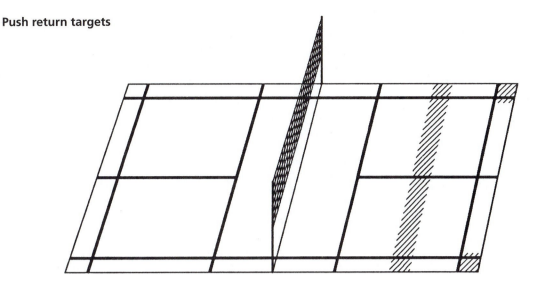

Serving and Scoring

In badminton only the server can score points. The receiver must win a rally in order to be able to serve and then have an opportunity to score.

In singles the serve is from the right service court whenever the server's score is an even number. The serve is from the left court whenever the server's score is an odd number. Remember that the service court for singles is long and narrow and that the sideline is the inside court boundary.

In doubles the serving team will always start an inning with the server in the right service court serving first. If the serving team wins the point, the same server moves to the left court and serves. The server keeps alternating courts until the serve is lost by a fault (see chapter 3).

When the first server has lost the serve in the first inning of play, the service is over, and the opponents serve. The team that serves first in doubles keeps the serve only as long as the original server continues to make points. (After the very first inning, each

player continues to serve until there is a fault.)

The opponents' first server will serve from the right court. If a point is made, he or she will move to the left court. Courts are alternated until the first server has lost the serve. The second server will then serve from the same court in which he or she was standing when the serve was lost. In other words, one cannot serve twice in a row to the same receiver. After the starting team has lost the service, the second team serving is allowed to have each server serve until the point is lost.

Once the original receivers have both lost their serves (called *two hands down*), the team that served first in the game will regain the serve. This time each player on that team must lose his or her serve before the other team gets another turn at serving.

A simple way to remember who should serve first in an inning is to recall which side of the court you were in during your team's first serve. You should be on that same side whenever your team's score is zero or an even number. You should be on the other side of the court whenever your team's score is an odd number.

The *rally* begins once the shuttle is served legally over the net, and it continues until one team has made a fault. If the serving team faults, the partner then takes the turn.

Once you begin to play, you will realize the importance of position, footwork, and strategy.

Summary

1. Only the person serving can score points, so the serve is very important.

2. The basic serves are the clear and the short, but a flick serve or a backhand serve can also be used. In singles, the high, deep serve is most often used; in doubles, the low, short serve. The drive serve is a change-up serve that can be very effective, as is the flick serve.

3. Whether playing singles or doubles, mix up your serves.

4. In singles the server serves from the right court whenever the server's score is an even number. The server serves from the left court whenever the score is an odd number.

5. In doubles the first inning allows only one player to serve. That player serves first from the right court and alternates sides with each point won. When the other team gains its serve, the server in the right court serves until his or her team has committed a fault. Then the partner serves. After each point, the server alternates courts.

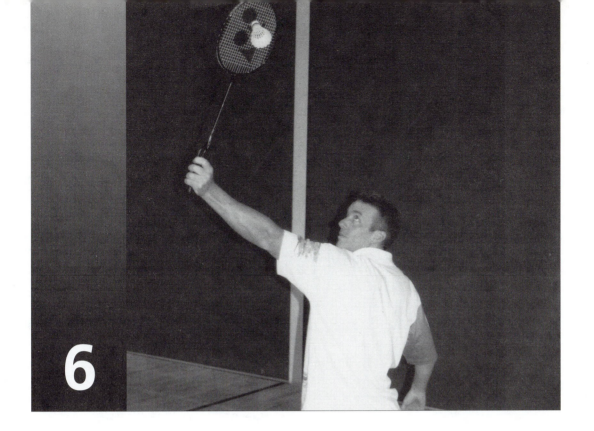

6

Overhead Strokes

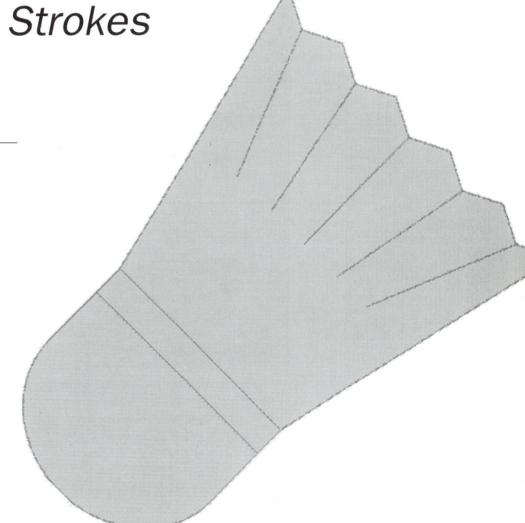

Chapter Outline

Basic overhead strokes:

A. Topview

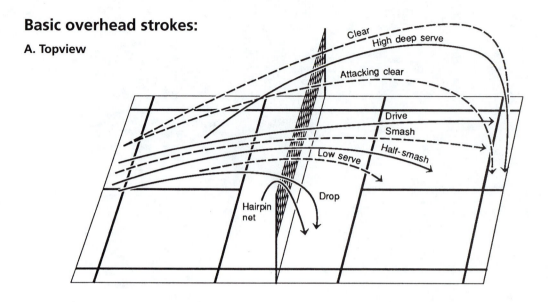

B. Sideview

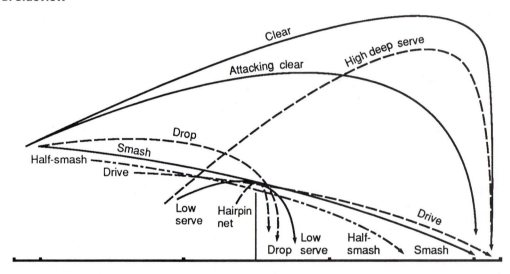

The overhead strokes that are absolutely essential for any badminton player are the clear, the smash and half-smash, drop, dab or push, and the drive. These are the "fun" strokes.

There are very few service aces in badminton. Most of the points come from rallies. Since the net is 5 feet high, you will want to hit most strokes above your head. This way you have the option of hitting downward hard or hitting a controlling shot that places the shuttle quickly in an area difficult for your opponent to cover.

If you are forced to hit underhand, your choices are limited, allowing your opponent to control the game. To be in control, you must play an attacking game by hitting as many overhead shots as possible, forcing your opponent to hit up or to hit from deep in the backcourt.

Forehand clear:

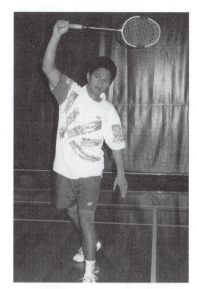

A. Backhand

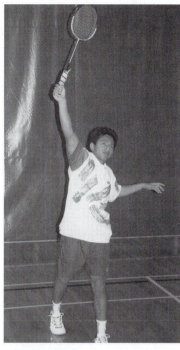

B. Foreswing

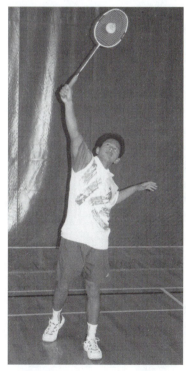

C. Contact

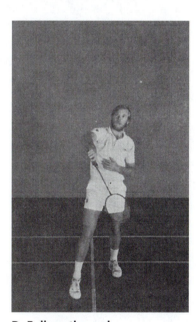

D. Follow-through

The fundamental overhead strokes for beginners are

- forehand and backhand clears and drops and
- forehand smash.

The intermediate-level overhead shots are

- drives and
- round-the-head shots.

The advanced overhead shots are

- backhand smash,
- attacking clear, and
- half-smash.

Forehand Overhead Clear

The *forehand overhead clear* is used mostly in singles to move an opponent to the backcourt. Take a forehand grip; then, from your base position, watch the oncoming shuttle and get into position behind it, with your right shoulder in line with it. Bring your racket up and behind your shoulders with the head pointing slightly downward. This is often called the "back-scratching" position because the racket head is nearly touching your back. Get into this position quickly. If you hit the shuttle while you are moving backward, you are not getting back and behind the shuttle quickly enough.

When you hit this shot, your left shoulder should be closest to the net and your left arm extended and pointing up at the shuttle. Your weight will shift to the right leg as you prepare for the shot and take your backswing, and then shift to the left foot as the stroke is taken.

Bring the racket up to meet the shuttle as high as possible. The shuttle is contacted above and in front of your shoulder, not out to the side. It is hit at the highest point possible. At contact, your arm straightens, and your forearm pronates and your wrist flexes. The racket head will be facing upward slightly at contact. Let the racket continue outward and to the left side of your body. When you shift your weight to your forward foot, keep your forward knee slightly flexed for balance.

The overhead clear shot should drop perpendicular to the floor and land between the baseline and the long doubles service line. This deep shot, which drops straight down, is more difficult for your opponent to hit. If you have time, look at your opponent's feet to see whether they are near the baseline, which is a good indication that your clear is deep.

You will note that the shuttle does not follow the same path as a ball would follow. A ball follows an arc path—with the angle of ascent and descent approximately the same. The shuttle, because it is so light and has great air speed, almost immediately slows down and then drops nearly straight down. Because of its unusual flight path, beginners often have trouble anticipating where the shuttle will drop.

A good clear will also give you more time to get back to home base (in the center of your court) and will make it more difficult for your opponent to smash effectively, because one cannot smash effectively from deep court. Remember to return to your home base and be in your ready position after each shot.

When you can hit the clear consistently, you may want to play a *long and short game*. In this game you will try to keep your opponent back most of the time while occasionally hitting a drop shot to break his or her rhythm.

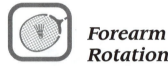

Forearm Rotation

To learn the arm action for overhead strokes, follow this drill. Start without your racket. Your intention is to throw the shuttle up and out as far as possible. This throwing action is very similar to that used in hitting the clear smash.

Turn your body, and face the sidelines with your left shoulder toward the net. With your left foot forward (for right-handers) and

---

Checklist for the High Clear Shot

1. Are you in the ready position?
2. Do you have a forehand grip?
3. Are you behind the shuttle with your left shoulder pointing to it?
4. Is your racket pointed downward behind your back with your wrist cocked?
5. As you swing upward, do you contact the shuttle in front of your body with a forearm rotation and wrist flexion, hitting the shuttle high?
6. Do you follow through completely?

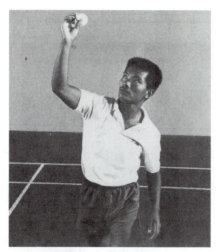

Throwing drill

weight on your back foot, take the shuttle in your right hand and hold it at the base. Bring your right elbow to shoulder height and away from your body. Your hand and the shuttle should be behind your right ear. Your wrist should be flexed toward the thumb side of your hand. Now throw the shuttle *up and out* as far as you can reach.

Transfer your weight to your forward (left) foot as you release the shuttle. Your upper torso will rotate to your left as your arm comes upward and forward. Try

throwing a few more times to get the overall sensation. Check your release in relation to your body with your best throws. This is the angle at which you want your racket to contact the shuttle.

Practice hint: Occasionally while rallying, have the opposite player let the shuttle drop so that you can see whether it lands near the base-line. This is where a good defensive clear should fall.

Hint for advanced players: To get back to the center of the court quickly, advanced players should "scissor" their legs as they hit the high clear shot. In this technique the weight is shifted from the racket-side leg to the other leg as the shuttle is hit. The player gets under the shuttle, jumps upward from the racket-side leg, and then, after hitting the shuttle, lands on the other leg and moves forward toward the home-base position.

Backhand clear:

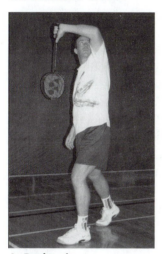

A. Backswing

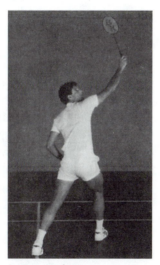

B. Foreswing

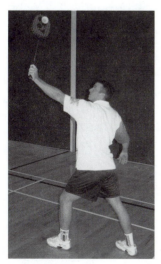

C. Contact

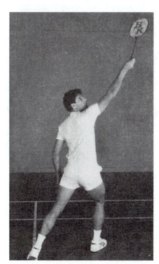

D. Follow-through

Backhand Overhead Clear

The *backhand overhead clear* is used mainly in singles when the player cannot get in position to hit a forehand. Always make the round-the-head shot if possible. Your back should be facing the net and your right foot pointed diago-nally toward the backhand corner of the court. Your elbow should be pointing up at the incoming shut-tle, and your wrist should be cocked. With elbow leading, supinate your forearm so your knuckles face the net and the racket head is whipped up to and through the incoming shuttle. The contact point is high and must be either in front or behind the shoulder. Your weight will shift to your right foot as you hit and follow through.

Attacking clear:

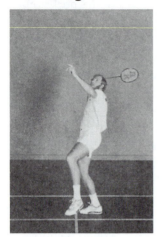

A. Backswing

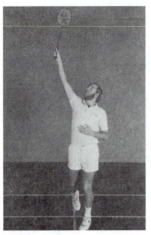

B. Foreswing

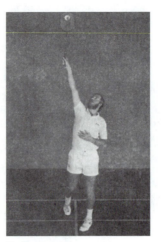

C. Contact

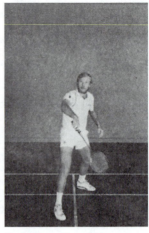

D. Follow-through

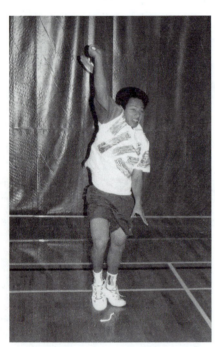

Footwork for scissors kick in smash

Attacking Clear

The *attacking clear* is used when your opponent is close to the net, and you think you can get the shuttle over his or her head. It is hit like a clear except that the trajectory is flatter and faster.

Smash

The *smash* is the most powerful stroke in badminton. It is hit extreme and, if hit effectively, usually ends the rally. However, speed is not as important as the downward angle.

Body position is the same as that for the clear, with one difference being in the angle of the racket at the contact point. In the clear the racket head is pointed up, while in the smash it is angled down. A second difference is the increased speed of your forearm and wrist snap.

As you get set for the smash, your left shoulder should be closest to the net. The shuttle should be ahead of your hitting shoulder—much farther ahead than where you contact the clear. (The weaker your wrist, the farther forward the shuttle should be hit.) You should hit the shuttle in front of your shoulder and at the highest point possible. Your shoulder, forearm, and wrist will rotate rapidly forward as the shuttle is contacted. Hitting it slightly ahead of your body will give you a greater sharpness of angle on the shot.

As you hit the smash, your upper body should move forward and downward. This facilitates power and follow-through. If you are behind the middle of the court, your forward momentum helps you to get back into the home-base position more quickly and get set for a possible return.

The smash should land near either sideline and at approximately midcourt—10 to 16 feet from the net.

Use this shot only when you expect it to be a winner. Since you will be expending a great deal of energy and may be off balance after your follow-through, it is important that it be done effectively.

Backhand smash:

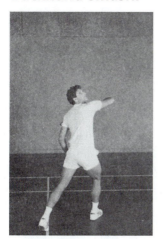 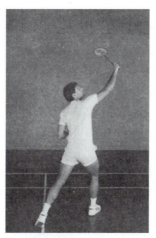 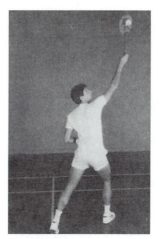 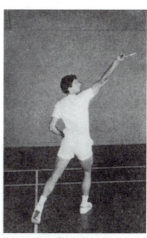

| A. Backswing | B. Foreswing | C. Contact | D. Follow-through |

The smash should be used only when you are in the front three-quarters of the court unless you are a very strong player. Beyond that area your opponent will probably have time to return it, because the shuttle will lose speed as it flies the greater distance, and your opponent can see the shuttle for a longer period of time. But if you have a chance to hit a smash when you are in the forecourt area, there is a very good chance that it will be a winner.

If you find that you are smashing into the net, it means either that you are hitting the shuttle too far in front of you or that you have an exceptionally strong wrist snap. In either case, move under the shuttle a bit more, so that it is not so far in front of you before you hit it. If you are hitting out of bounds, you will need to hit the shuttle farther in front of your body or use more wrist snap.

The smash is probably the most overused stroke in the game—especially among younger players. The best strategy is almost always to move your opponent up and back, side to side, and wait patiently for the opening for a smash that will be a winner and end the rally.

You can occasionally hit a smash at your opponent's body. The chest-to-hip area on the racket-side of your opponent is most vulnerable to this type of shot.

 Checklist for the Smash

1. Are you facing the right sideline?
2. Is your racket pointed down behind your back in the backswing?
3. Do you swing high and then contact the shuttle in front of your body with a hard, downward wrist snap?
4. Do you shift your weight to your left foot as you complete a full follow-through?

Half-smash:

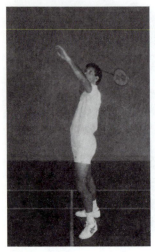 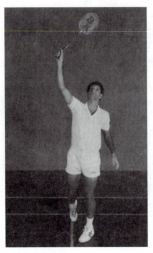 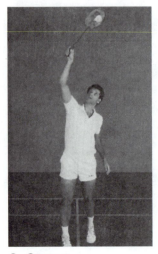 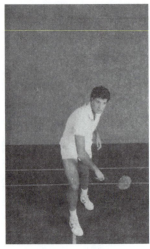

A. **Backswing**   B. **Foreswing**   C. **Contact**   D. **Follow-through**

**Half-smash trajectories
and targets**

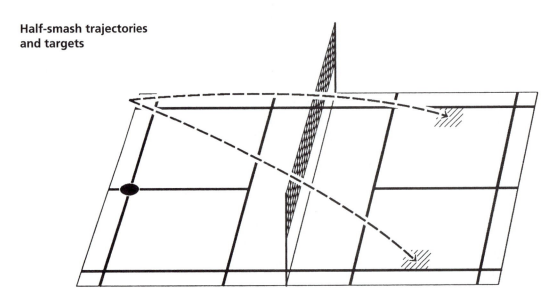

Half-Smash

The *half-smash* is an attacking stroke used in singles, doubles, and mixed doubles. It is hit similarly to the smash, but placement rather than speed is essential. The power will come more from the wrist snap than from the whole body.

This shot provides a good change of pace. It is essential to place it to the side of the court and with a sharp downward trajectory so that your opponent cannot reach it.

The half-court smash, which lands about midcourt, is often more effective than the full smash, which may land deep in your opponent's backcourt. Actually, both shots should be used. When you play both, you keep your opponent guessing as to whether to move up or back to cover your shot.

Drop shot:

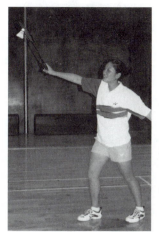

A. Backswing

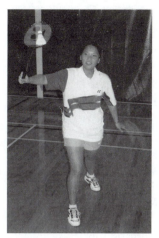

B. Foreswing

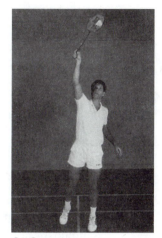

C. Contact

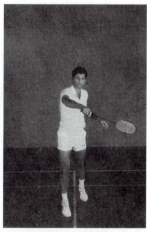

D. Follow-through

Drop shot

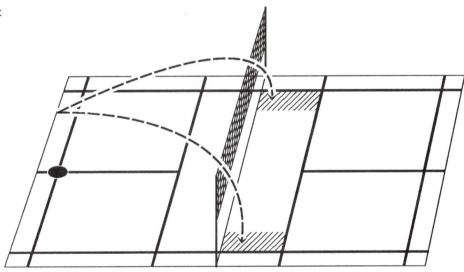

Drop Shot

The *drop shot* is a soft shot that barely clears the net and then lands close to the net on the other side—preferably in one of the front corners. It is used to move your opponent forward and to force an upward return that may give you the opportunity for a smash shot. It can be used effectively when your opponent is deep or expects a smash.

The arm action for the drop shot should look like the clear—and vice versa—so that you can disguise your shots and thereby surprise your opponent. Use the combination of clear and drop to move your opponent back and forward. This strategy will cause fatigue and will often keep him or her off balance. Remember that deception is the key.

In the drop shot, the shuttle is contacted in front of the body and the speed of the racket at the time of the hit is greatly slowed compared to the clear. The racket head

Dab:

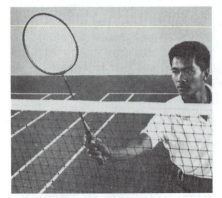

A. Foreswing

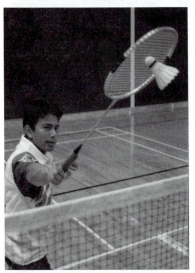

B. Contact

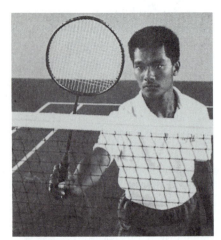

C. Follow-through

should be perpendicular to the floor or slightly past the perpendicular.

The swing speed should start fast to look like a clear or a smash, but the elbow and wrist snap should be slow as you softly guide the shuttle over the net with your follow-through. If you fail to disguise this shot, your opponent will be able to get the jump on you and make an easy play. Many beginners look like the Statue of Liberty, standing motionless during this shot—a dead giveaway.

Rather than arcing up and coming down, the trajectory of the shuttle should start immediately down from the racket and fall into your opponent's forecourt just past the net. The lower you have to reach to contact the shuttle, and the farther you have to hit it, the more you will have to open the face of the racket upward.

Drop shots can be hit very soft and land just past the net, or they can be hit harder, dropping a bit farther from the net. The softness of the shot will be determined by how much of the wrist snap you eliminate as you are contacting the shuttle and making your follow-through.

Push or Dab Shot

The *push* or *dab* is used at the net, primarily in doubles play. It is more of a sidearm block than an overhead shot, hit downward with little or no backswing. The elbow is flexed and held in front of the body. You lunge at the shuttle with your racket-side leg leading. The wrist does not uncock as you push the shuttle, and the follow-through will be very short. You are looking for placement rather than speed in this shot, the most effective placement being near midcourt, between the opponents, and to the sideline.

Timing is very important on the push stroke, which is used primarily in doubles. It is most effective against a team playing up and back.

Drive Shot

Drive shots are sidearm shots played from either the forehand or the backhand sides. These hard shots travel parallel to the net and are used to hit an opening your opponent has left or to force your opponent to quickly cover side to side.

Checklist for the Drop Shot

1. Do you make the shot look like a smash or a clear by swinging up hard?
2. Do you slow the speed of the racket just before contact to greatly reduce the wrist snap?
3. At contact, was the racket perpendicular to the floor?
4. Do you gently guide the shuttle over the net with your slow follow through?

Forehand drive:

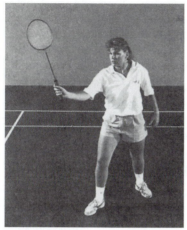

A. Foreswing

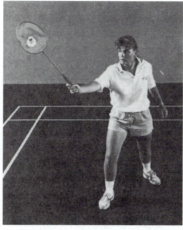

B. Contact

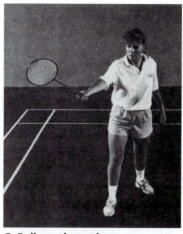

C. Follow-through

Backhand drive:

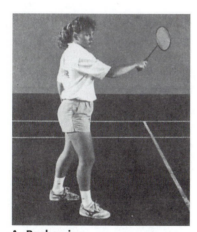

A. Backswing

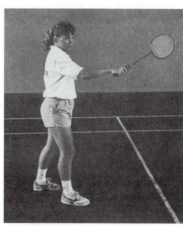

B. Foreswing

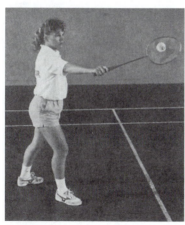

C. Contact

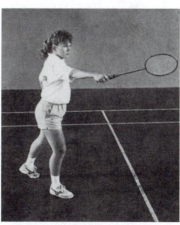

D. Follow-through

For the forehand drive, use your forehand grip and swing in a circular path, whipping your wrist as you contact the shuttle. The contact point is diagonally in front of your left foot. Play it at as high a point as possible so that you will not be hitting up at the shuttle.

Be sure that you are not crowding the shuttle by getting too close. You want to be able to swing freely at it. Your follow-through will be around your body. Your arm and racket will have completed about three-fourths of a circle.

For the backhand drive shot, you use a backhand grip and less wrist but more elbow movement. As you get set for the shot, turn your body so that you are facing the left sideline. Make your backswing with much more elbow bend than in the regular drive shot. Then, with your right elbow pointing at the oncoming shuttle, shift your weight to your right foot as you swing with your shoulders, arm, and wrist. Hit the shuttle in front of you, then follow through around your body.

Your drives can be played down the near sideline or

Round-the-head shot:

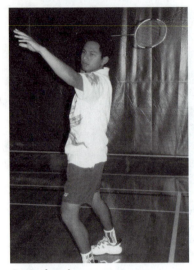

A. Backswing

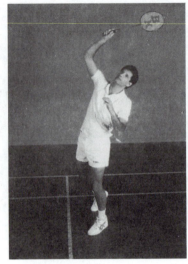

B. Foreswing

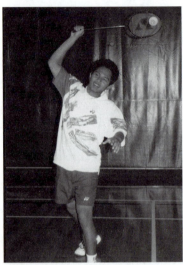

C. Contact

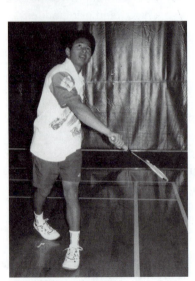

D. Follow-through

better height. The backswing is similar to that for other overhead shots, but the contact point is above your left shoulder.

If your feet are on the floor, your weight should be on the left foot. If you jump for the shot, you should scissor your legs (a *switch step*), getting your right leg forward, to allow you to get back to your home-base position more quickly.

crosscourt, depending on where your opponent has left an opening. Your shots should be hit hard, in a path parallel to the floor, just clearing the net. If your opponent is forced to play your drive while it is still moving fast, there is less likelihood of an effective return. And if it is not played quickly and begins to drop, your opponent will be forced to hit up, giving you the advantage here, too.

 ## Round-the-Head Shot

More advanced players often hit what is called a *round-the-head* shot. Clears, smashes, and drops can all be hit with this stroking action, which is done to avoid having to take a shot on the backhand side (a weaker or a defensive shot). A round-the-head shot allows you to stay on the attack.

Your grip will be a forehand grip—although some players prefer a frying-pan grip. The shot will be made with your body facing the net or while you are jumping to get

Summary

1. For all overhead strokes, the direction of the shuttle will be determined by the angle of the racket at the time of contact. So, when practicing, concentrate on which racket angle gives you the exact trajectory that you want.

2. Get behind the shuttle as quickly as you can to better enable you to make the kind of shot that you want to make.

3. Always try to take the offense when your opponent hits you a high shot—especially one that is high and short.

4. Always contact the shuttle as high as possible.

5. The major overhead shots are
   a. forehand overhead clear,
   b. backhand overhead clear,
   c. drop shot,
   d. smash,
   e. half-smash,
   f. dab or push,
   g. forehand drive,
   h. backhand drive, and
   i. round-the-head shots.

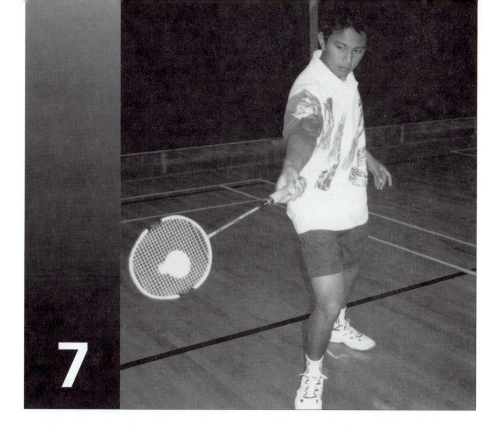

7

Underhand Strokes and Smash Returns

Chapter Outline

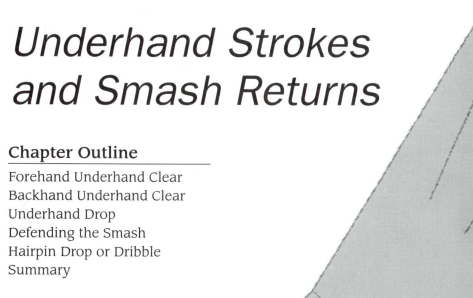

While you would prefer to hit all of your shots downward, using overhead strokes, your opponents will often catch you with a drop shot or smash, and then you will have to hit underhanded. In doing so, you will be playing a defensive game. You will therefore want to keep your opponent off balance by hitting the shuttle deep in a clearing shot or having the shuttle drop close to the net.

The underhand shots are

- underhand clear,
- underhand drop, and
- hairpin drop.

As in all badminton shots, you want to hit the shuttle at the highest point possible.

Forehand Underhand Clear

When your opponent makes an effective drop shot into your forecourt, you must go on the defensive, so it is best to hit an underhand clear. This will force your opponent into the backcourt and give you time to get back to your home-base position.

Assuming that the shuttle is dropping toward your forehand side, get to the shuttle as fast as you can. Your first step will be a short one with the left leg. Your right leg should then come forward with a long enough step to bring you to the shuttle.

Reach for the shuttle. Getting too close will inhibit your swing. Bring your racket down and under the oncoming shuttle. Your wrist should be slightly cocked. Make sure that your palm faces the ceiling. Keep your upper body and chin upright and keep the non-racket arm up and behind the body for balance.

Contact the shuttle in front of your body with your weight on your forward foot. Follow through with the arm to the nonracket shoulder. Lift the shuttle to the corner you intend the shuttle to go. Follow through in the direction that you intend the shuttle to go. It should land within 2 feet of your opponent's baseline, and its flight should resemble that of a high singles serve.

Remember to step with your right foot. This will extend your reach about 1 foot. It will also allow you to get back to your home base more quickly to get ready for the next shot.

On crosscourt shots, contact the shuttle harder to make up the extra distance it will have to travel.

Checklist for the Underhand Clear

1. Step to the shuttle with your right foot forward as you hit it.
2. Bring the racket head under the shuttle with your wrist cocked.
3. Hit hard, with a great deal of wrist action.
4. Follow through in your intended line of flight.

Forehand underhand clear:

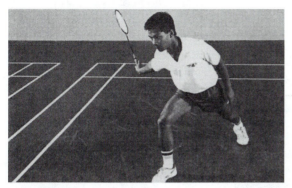

A. Backswing

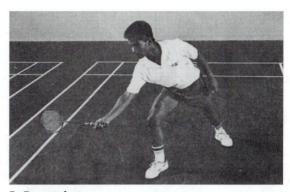

B. Foreswing

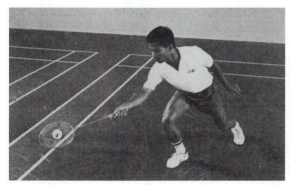

C. Contact

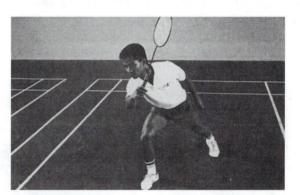

D. Follow-through

Backhand Underhand Clear

On strokes made from your non-racket side, change to a backhand grip. Your last step as you reach for the shuttle will be with your right foot. Get to the shuttle as soon as possible. Your racket should be in line with and behind the shuttle.

Lead with the elbow and extend the forearm and hand through the shuttle up to the racket shoulder. The shuttle should travel high and to the baseline area.

Underhand Drop

The underhand drop is played from behind the front service line. It is very similar to a low serve in that it should just clear the net and then drop quickly. This shot is valuable primarily in doubles play when played from midcourt. It can force a net player to move from side to side, or it can bring backcourt players to the net if they are playing side by side. In singles, it is generally used to return a smash, forcing the smashing player to cover some distance and then go on the defensive by hitting up.

Backhand underhand clear:

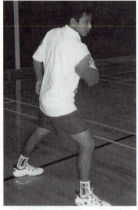
A. Backswing

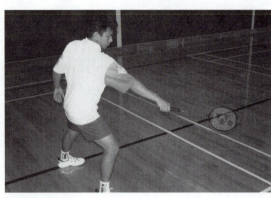
B. Foreswing

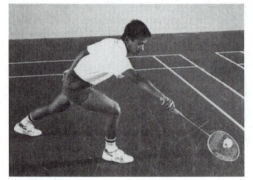
C. Contact

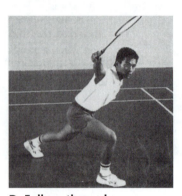
D. Follow-through

Defending the Smash

To defend against the smash, spread your legs, bend your knees, and keep the racket well in front of the body with the hand at least waist high. Once the smash is hit, watch the shuttle for its location and speed and move your racket forward to contact the shuttle. Your return may be sidearm or underhand stroke.

The *block shot* is like the *dab shot*. It should land close to the net. Since it requires no backswing, you can use it to make the return even if you just barely get to the smash. If you don't have time to aim it, just block it straight.

A backhand shot gives you a greater range of blocking area—from shots aimed from the racket side leg to the nonracket sideline. With a forehand you have a range from in front of your racket-side leg to the sideline on your racket side.

Your return of the smash should get the shuttle back to an area that is difficult for your opponent to cover. Keep your opponent off balance with a mix of drops, clears, and drives. Also, smashes must be returned quickly, or the speed of the shuttle will have it past you in an instant.

The quickness required for your smash returns will limit you to primarily wrist shots. You won't have time to wind up and take a full backswing. Also, keep your opponent guessing as to where you will return your shot.

In singles you will generally use a blocking action to return a smash, dropping the shuttle next to the net, an underhand drop, or a crosscourt block. In doubles you will generally use drive shots down the near sideline. For the blocks, simply get your racket in front of the shuttle, and let the speed of the smashed shuttle provide part of the power for the return. For the drive shots, you will have to supply some of the power needed with your wrist or arm.

On smashes aimed at the body, try to move your body away from the smash. It is easier to play a smash aimed at the backhand side of your body, because with the racket in your right hand, your hand will be farther from the shuttle. In any case, try to hit the shuttle as far in front of you as possible.

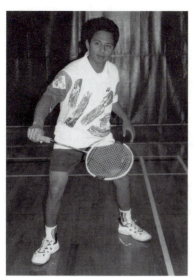

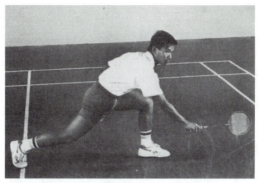

Backhand block of a smash

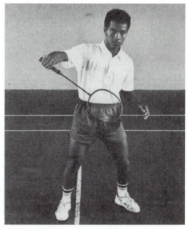

Blocking a smash at the body

zDefending a smash by dropping the racket head low

 ## *Hairpin Drop or Dribble*

The hairpin drop is played after your opponent has hit a tight drop shot close to the net. The idea is to guide the shuttle gently over the top of the net and have it drop as close to the net as possible.

Get to the shuttle quickly, so that you can contact the shuttle as close to the top of the net as possible. In singles you don't have to be quite as precise with your placement as you do in doubles.

Your grip should be loose. Step toward the shuttle with your racket-side foot. The stroke is executed with your forearm and wrist. With elbow at chest height and the racket in front and to side of body, the extension of the forearm will guide the shuttle over the net gently.

You can place the shuttle directly in front of where you contact it, or you can guide it to a front corner of the court. Its flight path will be determined by the angle of your racket head at the point of contact.

Keep the shuttle close to the top of the net so that it cannot be smashed back at you. It should just clear the net and then drop, making it very difficult to return.

In doubles, with one person playing up and one back, you will be closer to the shuttle on this type of shot—but so is your opponent. You will have more area next to the net toward which to aim. You will need more variation and deception in your technique in order to hit safely to any spot forecourt. For that reason, when playing doubles you may want to *choke* up on your grip a bit (slide your hand up the handle) for better control.

 Checklist for the Hairpin Drop

1. Hold the racket loosely with a forehand grip.
2. Step with the right foot toward the shuttle.
3. Gently guide the shuttle over the net—as close to the top of the net as possible.

Hairpin drop:

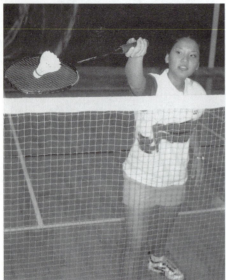

A. Contact

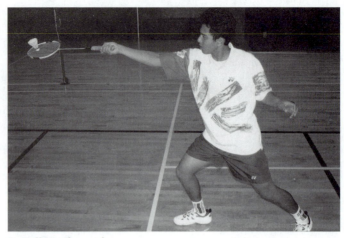

B. Follow-through

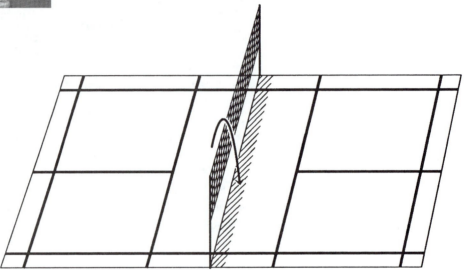

Summary

1. While it is always preferable to hit with an overhead stroke, a good opponent will force you to hit many shots under-handed.

2. Always try to use your under-hand shot to get your opponent off balance and to force a return to you that is high and short.

3. An effective drop shot at the net forces your opponent to hit the shuttle up. This may give you a setup for a smash or a drive.

4. A high clear to your opponent can put him or her on the defensive.

5. One of the most effective shots to counter your opponent's drop is the dribble or hairpin drop.

6. On smash returns, block the shuttle as far in front of you as possible.

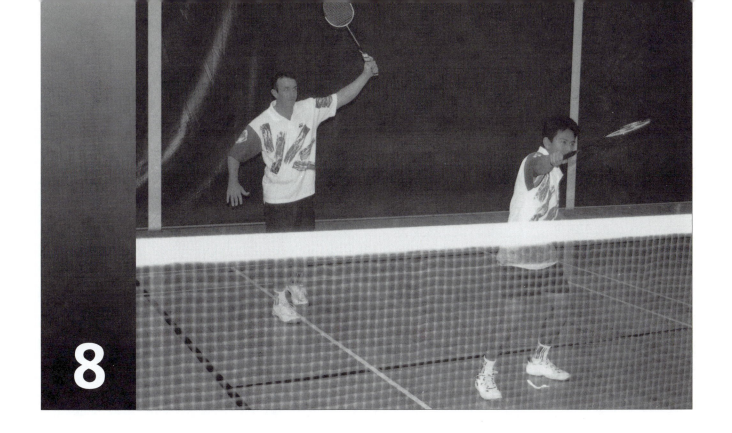

8

Strategy

Chapter Outline

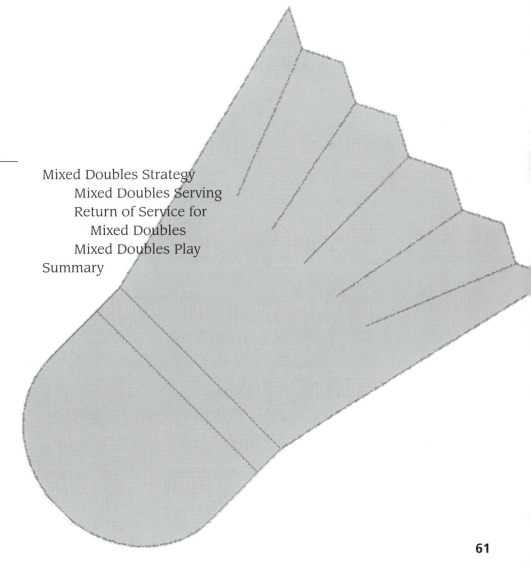

One of the major thrills of badminton is outsmarting your opponent. Wise strategic decisions, if properly executed with good fundamentals, will win many games. As you gain experience and expertise, you will have more strategic options. In this chapter we will look at strategy from the beginning level to the more advanced levels.

Basic Strategy

1. Keep the shuttle away from your opponent.

2. Move your opponent out of the center of the court (the home-base position).

3. When in doubt, place the shuttle behind your opponent and hope for a weak return.

4. The backhand is usually the weaker side, so play to that.

5. While it is obvious that a left-hander's backhand is the same side as a right-hander's forehand, people often forget this. Remember to avoid hitting toward the forehand of a left-handed opponent under the mistaken notion that it is his or her backhand.

6. Move toward the center of the court after each shot (home base).

7. Use the smash to finish rallies, not as a basic shot to move your opponent and create openings.

Your Fundamental Shots

Good strategic decisions are wasted without good fundamentals. Remember these key points:

■ Try always to hit the shuttle at as high a point as possible and as

soon as possible. Don't wait for the shuttle to come to you. Move to it quickly and get behind it.

■ Deception is a key element in this game, so you should attempt to make your strokes look similar as long as possible. For example, when a shot is hit high, you can fake a drop and hit a clear, or fake a smash and hit a drop.

Developing Game Strategy during Warm-up

Try out various shots on your opponent during warm-up to see how he or she reacts to them. Especially try (1) drops to check your opponent's speed and ability and (2) clears to the backhand side to check on his or her strength there—and also to see whether he or she runs around the backhand, thereby opening up an area to the forehand side.

Note whether your opponent seems slow or lazy. Is there a pattern to his or her returns, such as always hitting straight or crosscourt, or always clearing or dropping? Does your opponent want to smash too often, even when out of position or off balance? These observations will help you plan your strategy.

If you are in a tournament, watch your future opponents in their matches to discover their strengths and weaknesses.

Target areas for singles

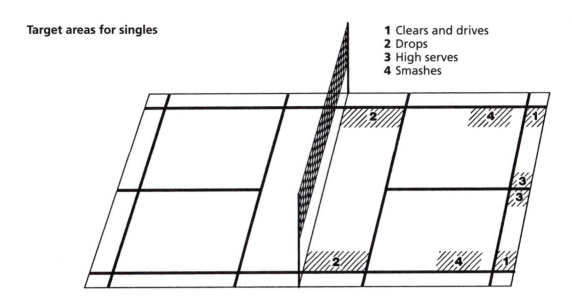

1 Clears and drives
2 Drops
3 High serves
4 Smashes

Singles Strategy

Most of your singles serves will be high and deep (whereas most of your doubles serves will be low and short). Throw in some flicks and drives, but mix them up so that your opponent cannot antici- pate them. Try to be deceptive on your serves as well as on your strokes. And remember that if your serves are fast, the returns from your opponent are likely to be fast, so be ready for them.

Singles Serving

Singles serving is usually a high, deep shot to the back of the court near the midline. By serving near the midline of the backcourt, you cut down angle that your opponent can hit. But, again, vary your serves so that your opponent can- not guess exactly what you will do.

Once you've established the high, deep serve to the midline, observe your opponent's pattern of service returns. Use the short serve and the flick serve for variety, again aiming near the midline.

If your opponent is playing a bit too deep, hit a short serve. And if he or she is playing too close, hit the high, clear serve. Watch for evidence that one particular serve gives your opponent trouble.

Return of Service for Singles

At the beginning level, at least 80 percent of your returns should be straight ahead. Usually a clear or drop down the line would be good choices to start the rally. Your service return should move your opponent out of the center court position—this will open up the entire court for your next shot.

The only time you would use a smash on a service return is on a high, short serve. Even then, use the smash only if you are certain that you can "put the bird on the floor." If you try to smash an effective serve, you will probably hit too flat and be off-balance for the reply (return) and will quickly be the one at a disadvantage.

The returns you'll use most often for a high serve are a high clear or a drop in the near corner away from your opponent. If a high serve is short (in front of the back doubles service line) you may smash, hit an attacking clear, or a drop to either near corner. If your opponent serves short and low, your best returns are a drop to the near corner or a flick or attacking clear, provided your opponent is close to the front service line.

Singles Rally Strategy

A primary rule of rally strategy is that whenever you get in trouble, you should hit the clear to your opponent's backhand. This gives you time to recover and may force your opponent into a weak return.

If you can get your opponent moving forward and backward, you will have an advantage. Try to move him or her into the various corners of the court and away from the controlling position in the center of the court. By moving your opponent, you may force weak returns and create holes in his or her defense. For you to keep control of the rally, you must maintain your strong position at your home base.

A popular combination is a clear to the backhand, then a drop to the forehand, followed by another deep backhand clear and another forehand drop. This makes your opponent move a great distance and execute a weak shot (the high backhand) at the end of a long run.

With a continued pattern of clears and drops, you will eventually force your opponent to hit a weak return. This is the time for you to win the point with a smash. You must have both patience and endurance for this defensive type of strategy. Once you get your opponent moving, you can take the offensive. Vary your shots. You can hit a hard drive or a smash directly at your opponent as he or she charges the net. If your opponent runs quickly forward after you have hit a clear, you might hit two clears in a row. You can then hit a drive behind your opponent as he or she is moving in the opposite direction.

While every player should be adept at both offensive shots and defensive shots, before starting serious training you should determine whether you want to emphasize the offensive or defensive aspects of your game. Which style fits you best?

If you are strong and can hit hard, you may opt to be an attacking player. If you are quick, have stamina, and perhaps are shorter than average, you might choose to play a more defensive game. In either case you will need to practice all of your fundamentals, because the offensive players will use many clears and drops, and the defensive players will sometimes use the smash.

To defend a smash, block it, and drop it close to the net. If your opponent has smashed straight, you might drop it crosscourt. If he or she has smashed crosscourt, drop it in the near front corner.

If you are trailing your opponent's score late in a game, you might switch your strategy to a safer one called the *center court theory,* in which you avoid the sidelines in your shots. Hit smashes at your opponent's body —between the waist and shoulder of the racket side of the body. Such a strategy reduces your chance of hitting the shuttle out of bounds, and it reduces the angle of return by your opponent. (*Note:* This is an exception to the badminton courtesy of avoiding hits into the body of an opponent as a common practice.)

Checklist for Singles Strategy

1. Move your opponent from the home-base position to the corners.
2. Force your opponent to hit up (play defensively) as often as possible.
3. Hit deep, especially to the backhand, to force weak returns.
4. Hit the shuttle as early and as high as possible.
5. Disguise your shots and vary them.
6. When returning smashes, hit deep or short—never to the midcourt area.

Block, straight, smash cross-court

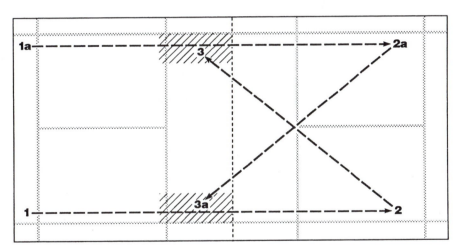

Block, cross-court, smash, straight

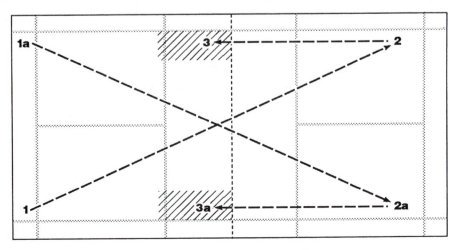

Target areas for doubles:

1 Low serves
2 Flicks and drive serves
3 Drop shots
4 Drives and smashes
5 Half smashes and pushes

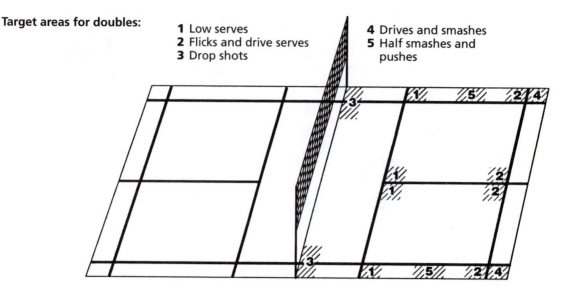

Doubles Strategy

Doubles is a more complex game than singles. It demands faster reactions and being able to anticipate what your partner and your opponents will do with the shuttle. Good doubles play begins with an effective serve or service return (the most important parts of the game) and ends with good teamwork on offense.

Doubles Serving

The server in a doubles game must vary the placement of the serve to prevent the opponent from attacking the serve. The short serve, the drive, and the high flick serves are used in doubles. The low, short serve to the near corner (the diagonal **T** area) is the most common serve. Top-caliber servers can often make points with a shot that is generally thought to be defensive.

Deception, an essential in the game of badminton, is particularly important in the serve. Make certain that the beginning of your serving action is the same for every type of serve you execute.

Return of Service for Doubles

The return for beginners should start with the ready position taken a few feet back from the front service line. As you become advanced, you will move up to within one foot of the front service line and within one foot of the centerline. From this point any low serves can be played quickly and at a high point.

Drop returns should be played straight ahead, not crosscourt. Drive returns should be at the backhand or down the near sideline. Push returns should be at the near sideline and to midcourt.

The best service returns for doubles are

- a push along the near sideline to midcourt,
- a drop shot away from the server's side,
- a drive to the deep corner on the near side,
- a push shot just behind the server, or
- a push into the body of the server's partner.

Target areas for doubles return:

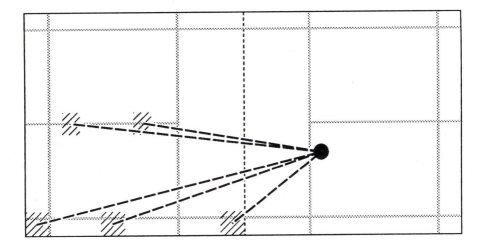

Defensive Strategy for Doubles

Effective service, service return, and rallies in doubles play all begin with proper alignment. Start your play from the best position for what you want to accomplish. You can play a defensive alignment (*side by side*), an offensive alignment (*up and back*), or you can use a combination of these two formations (*circular rotation*), depending on the situation.

In the *side-by-side alignment*, the basic defensive position for doubles, each partner is responsible for his or her half of the court. This alignment is easy to learn and eliminates confusion as to who will take a shot.

The defender directly in front of the attacker takes all shuttles that are hit to the sideline, all drop shots to his or her side of the court, all shots at the body, and all the high clears down the middle. The partner, who turns slightly toward the attacker, takes all the smashes hit to the center of the court or crosscourt and all drop shots on his or her side of the court.

This side-by-side alignment makes it much more difficult for your opponents to smash effectively. A drawback, however, is that it allows your opponents to continue to play to the weaker partner, not only obtaining weaker returns but also tiring him or her. Also, as a defensive rather than an offensive formation, it reduces a team's chance to attack, and doubles is an offensive game.

To get back on offense, a team using this alignment should block its opponents' smashes into the half-court area or clear them crosscourt. The attacker should be forced to run sideways to maintain his or her attack. This way he or she will not be able to hit deep, angled smashes, and hence the defenders will have a better chance of playing half-court returns and getting back on offense.

Side-by-side alignment is the best strategy when your opponents are in control. However, it should be remembered that attacking (offensive strategy) rather than defending is generally the best plan for winning at doubles.

Side-by-side alignment for doubles

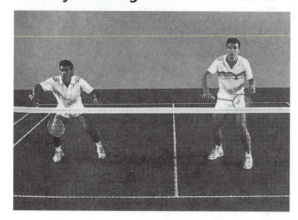
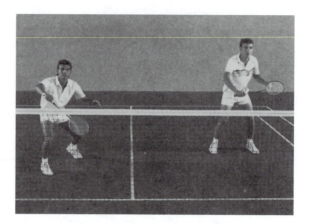

Basic side-by-side doubles alignment, with each player responsible for his or her half-court

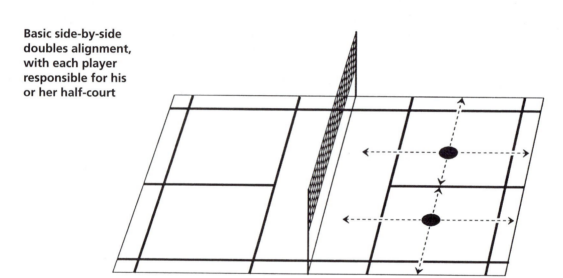

1 is responsible for shaded area.
2 is responsible for the unshaded area.

A is the attacker.

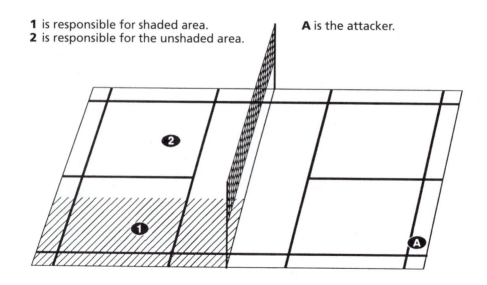

1 is responsible for unshaded area.
2 is responsible for the shaded area.

A is the attacker.

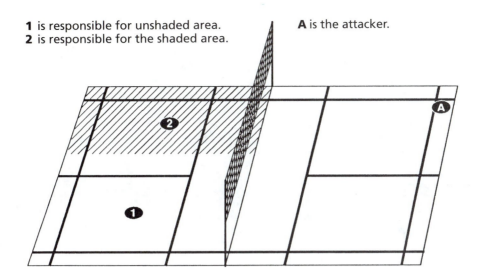

Offensive Strategy for Doubles

The *up-and-back alignment* for offensive play places both players in the midline of the court with one player close to the net, about one foot behind the **T** (the intersection of the midline and the short service line) and the other playing deep. This alignment (also easy to learn) is more effective against a team that hits strong, deep clears and short drops. One of its advantages is that the weaker player can be "hidden" at the net, with the stronger player playing most of the court. Another is that it is an attacking formation. Disadvantages are that the sides of the court are open to the smash and your opponents can run the backcourt player from side to side to tire him or her.

The normal pattern is for the server to play the "up" position after serving. The person receiving will play up if the serve is short and will play deep if the serve is long—with the partner playing the opposite position. In more advanced doubles, the stronger person will generally play deep and the weaker person up.

Both players must keep the shuttle low to the opponents. Any time that the shuttle is hit high, the net player becomes a sitting duck for a smash.

When playing the up-and-back alignment, if you are the up player, do not turn and look toward your partner. Keep your eyes on your opponents. There are two reasons for this recommendation. One is that you can get hit in the face with your partner's shot. The other is that by watching your opponents, you will know where the shuttle is going and will be able to adjust to its return more quickly.

The deeper player should adjust his or her position by playing slightly to the other side of the court from the up person. So if the up player is forced to the right, the back player will move to the left.

The success of offensive doubles depends to a large degree on the person playing near the net. This player can block shots and drop them close to the net, forcing the opponents into weak returns. Most rallies in good doubles are won by the net player.

The net player should take a position 1½ to 2 feet behind the

Up-and-back alignment for doubles

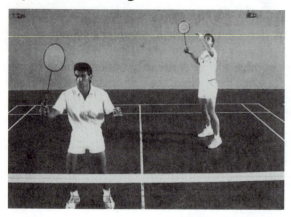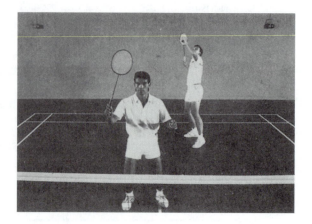

short service line. The racket should be held near net level. From this position you can move side to side and cut off most short shots. On a smash the forecourt player should defend the opposite side of the court from where the attacker is. This means that the forecourt player moves away from the centerline and back behind the short service line (see diagram).

From this position, the forecourt player should be able to make downward shots that the attackers will have to pop up. If it is not possible to hit the shuttle down, it should be blocked near the net to keep the opponents on the defensive.

The backcourt player should attempt to hit smashes down the line, into the center of the court, or into the body of the opponent who is nearest. The speed and angle of the smash should be varied to keep the opponents off-balance. Power is not as important in winning at doubles as variety and consistency.

Partners should be able to adjust to each other and to the expected shots of their opponents. For example, if the net player has hit a drop shot, the backcourt player can move up, expecting that the opponents will counter with another drop shot.

Experienced players will be able to see whether their opponents have moved forward or are too far back. They can then adjust their shots to take advantage of the resulting openings. Players who have played together for a long time will learn their partners' strengths and weaknesses and be able to set up their partners so that they make strong shots.

Combination Strategy

A combination of the side-by-side and up-and-back strategies is possible for more advanced players. As you get to know your partner, you can switch between side-by-side and up-and-back formations. Usually, if you hit the shuttle down, as in a drop, smash, or drive, you will go on offense and play up and back. If you lift the shuttle, you will likely go on defense and play side-by-side. A lower-level player may use verbal signals to alert the partner to a change, but advanced players learn to react to the proper position depending on the shot.

**Up-and-back doubles
alignment and court
responsibilities**

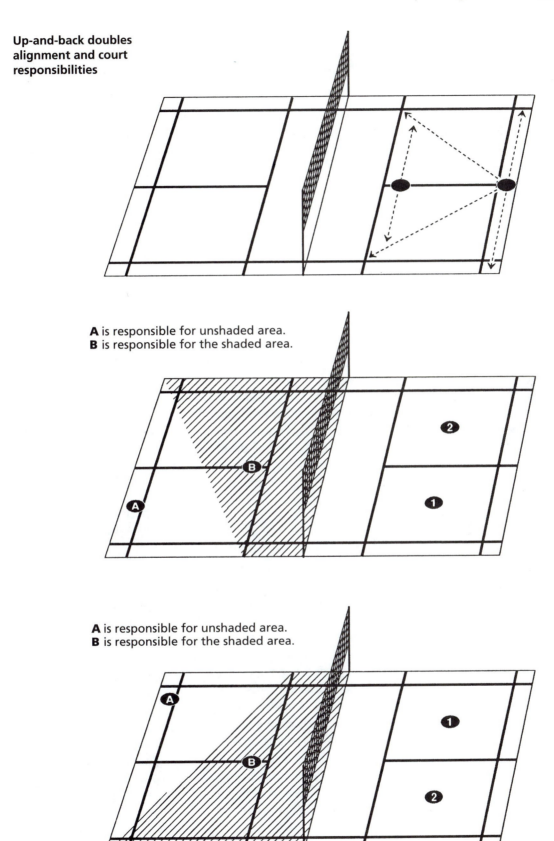

A is responsible for unshaded area.
B is responsible for the shaded area.

A is responsible for unshaded area.
B is responsible for the shaded area.

Checklist for Doubles Strategy

1. Against an up-and-back team
   a. Play to the weaker opponent.
   b. Hit shots to the corners to make opponents move up and back.
2. Against a side-by-side team
   a. Hit midcourt level shots to the sidelines.
   b. Hit shots to the corners to make opponents move sideways and to hit weaker returns or hit up.
   c. Smash to the sidelines as often as possible.

Mixed Doubles Strategy

At the championship level, men are generally stronger, taller, and faster than women. In physical education classes, these differences may not exist. For this reason, mixed doubles strategy will be discussed here in terms of the stronger and weaker player rather than the man and the woman.

Mixed Doubles Serving

The basic serve in mixed doubles is the short serve. However, doubles players should also have an effective flick serve in order to be able to take advantage of any weaknesses in the opponents' alignment or fundamental skills.

The short serve is usually served to the **T** (the intersection of the front service line with the midline.) A wide short serve to the side of the court is usually not employed because the down-the-line return of serve is simple to execute and difficult to defend against.

A flick serve can be used more often against the shorter and weaker (and therefore probably slower) player, from the usual

position at the net. It may also create gaps in the defense and allow the serving team to "put the bird on the floor."

The weaker player, who will be covering the shots close to the net, will serve from close to the front service line. The stronger player may serve from a deeper position to be ready for a high, clear return.

Return of Service for Mixed Doubles

The return of service is very important in mixed doubles. If the serve is poor (i.e., too high at the net), the receiver should move quickly to hit the shuttle down. The best return is usually straight back into the server at waist level and into the racket side of the body.

If the stronger player serves short and tight to the weaker opponent, the returner can make a net return to the sideline. A crosscourt net return might be intercepted by the opposing net player. Other times the shuttle can be pushed into the deep corners of the court before the stronger player is able to get back to cover them.

Block, cross-court, smash, straight:

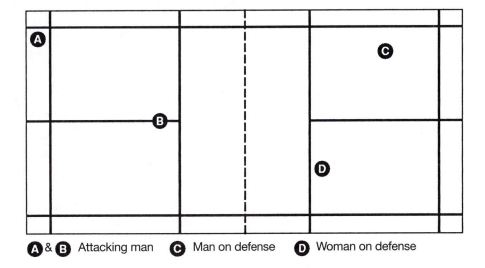

(A)&(B) Attacking man   (C) Man on defense   (D) Woman on defense

If the weaker player is serving to the weaker player on the other team, the returns should be straight ahead or dropped into the corner away from the server. Any crosscourt returns can be intercepted by the server and hit downward.

Short returns to the outside corners should be returned straight, regardless of who is serving.

In high-level competition, when the stronger player returns a serve from the weaker opponent, the shuttle should be pushed into the face or body of the weaker opponent. Another effective return is the half-court push to the sidelines. Avoid making a net shot straight ahead, because it can be cleared quickly over the stronger player's head, forcing the weaker partner to go into the backcourt.

When the stronger player returns service from an opposing strong player, the shuttle should be pushed to the sidelines at about half-court depth. It is most important for the stronger player to hit the return downward. After the return, the stronger player should move quickly to the backcourt to protect that area. The strongest alignment in mixed doubles is to have the weaker player up and the stronger player back. This puts the team in the best offensive position.

When either partner receives a flick serve, it should be smashed to the sidelines or into the server's body. Once in a while a fast drop or half-smash at the alley can be attempted.

Mixed Doubles Play

The play in mixed doubles should be concentrated toward the sidelines because the partners will be generally playing up and back. The shuttle should be hit down to make the opponents hit upward.

If you are forced to hit a high, clear shot, move into a *wedge formation,* because your opponents will probably hit a smash. In the wedge formation the stronger player aligns in front of the smasher and fairly deep in the court. The responsibility is for all shots to that side of the court. The weaker player defends the other

Checklist for Mixed Doubles Strategy

1. Play to the near sidelines.
2. Move the net player from side to side.
3. Try to hit every shot down.
4. Most serves should be low.

side of the court and aligns shorter to take crosscourt and midcourt shots and drops. The racket should be held in front of the body, with the head of the racket at head height.

Try to move the net player, usually the weaker player, from side to side with fast drops and crosscourt net shots. The shuttle should be played flat and directed down the sidelines. Crosscourt flat shots can be easily cut off by the opposing net player. However, if the deep player wants to hit a crosscourt shot, it should be hit over the head of the opposing net player to push him or her into the backcourt.

The net player, in general, should not try to intercept the straight half-court pushes unless he or she is certain of a good return. The net player should be content playing a good net game by hitting low net shots—not by hitting clears. When the shuttle is returned a bit higher than the top of the net, it should be smashed. The net player should hit every shot down, whether it be a drop, a drive, or a push.

On defense a wedge formation can be used when you have hit a high, weak return and expect a smash. The weaker player moves back a few steps and takes a position to intercept crosscourt smashes and drops. The smashes should be blocked away from the opposing net player.

Summary

1. Simple strategy includes
   a. keeping the shuttle away from your opponent;
   b. moving your opponent from the home-base position; and
   c. when in doubt, hitting a high clear to your opponent's backhand.
2. Singles serving strategy is based on serving mostly high, deep serves to the midline.
3. Singles strategy is designed to keep your opponent away from the home-base position.
4. The smash is the most over-used stroke in badminton.
5. Doubles is a more complex game than singles.
6. The serve is the most important part of a doubles game. Serves should be short and low or higher flick serves. Keep your opponent off balance.
7. The side-by-side alignment is a defensive formation.
8. The up-and-back alignment is an offensive formation.

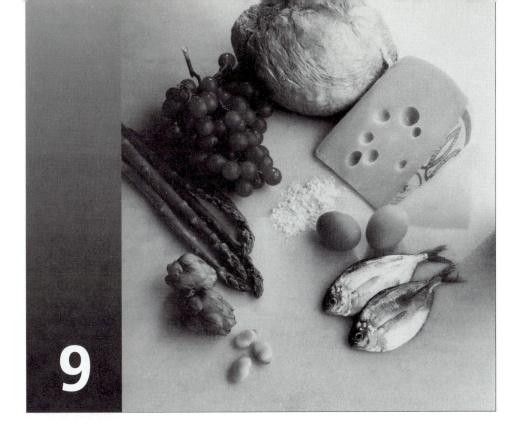

Increasing Your Physical and Mental Potentials

While most of this book deals with playing badminton, to live fully we must also be aware of our physical and mental conditioning. A long and full life requires exercise, an adequate diet, and play—both physical and mental. If you are going to play aggressive badminton, you will need adequate fuel for your athletic body, so let's start with nutrition.

Nutrition

A basic understanding of the science of nutrition is essential to healthy living. An informed person will be aware of the nutrients necessary for minimal function and then put that knowledge into practice by developing a proper diet. Unfortunately, very few of our citizens consume even the minimum amounts of each of the necessary nutrients: protein, fat, and carbohydrates, called the *macronutrients;* vitamins, minerals, and phytochemicals, called the *micronutrients;* and water, the essential nonnutrient.

The *calorie* used in counting food energy is really a kilocalorie, 1,000 times larger than the calorie used as a measurement of heat in chemistry class. In one food calorie (kilocalorie), there is enough energy to heat 1 kilogram of water 1 degree Celsius or to lift 3,000 pounds of weight one foot high. So those little calories you see listed on the cookie packages pack a lot of energy.

Most people need about 10 calories per pound just to stay alive. If you plan to do something other than just lie in bed all day, you may need about 17 calories per pound of body weight per day in order to keep yourself going.

Protein

Protein is made up of 22 amino acids composed of carbon, hydrogen, oxygen, and nitrogen. While both fats and carbohydrates contain the first three elements,

Muscle-Maintenance Program of 20 Calories (Kilocalories) per Pound				
Body Weight (Pounds)	Calories per Day	Calories from Carbohydrate (70%)	Calories from Protein (13–16%)	Calories from Fat (12–16%)
140	2800	2000	360–460	340–440
200	4000	2800	510–660	540–690

Muscle-Building Program of 25 to 30 Calories (Kilocalories) per Pound				
Body Weight (Pounds)	Calories per Day	Calories from Carbohydrate (70%)	Calories from Protein (13–16%)	Calories from Fat (12–16%)
140	3500–4200	2450–2940	455–670 (90–115 g per day)	420–672
200	5000–6000	3500–4200	650–960 (130–165 g per day)	600–960

The Essential Amino Acids and Some Foods That Contain Them

- Isoleucine: Fish, beef, organ meats, eggs, shellfish, whole wheat, soya, milk.
- Leucine: Beef, fish, organ meats, shellfish, eggs, soya, milk, liver.
- Lysine: Fish, beef, organ meats, shellfish, eggs, soya, milk, liver.
- Methionine: Fish, beef, shellfish, eggs, milk, liver, whole wheat, cheese.
- Phenylalanine: Beef, fish eggs, whole wheat, shellfish, organ meats, soya, milk.
- Threonine: Fish, beef, organ meats, eggs, shellfish, soya, liver.
- Tryptophan: Soy milk, fish, beef, soy flour, organ meats, shell fish, eggs.
- Valine: Beef, fish, organ meats, eggs, soya, milk, whole wheat, liver.

Amino Acid Requirements[a]

Amino Acid	Mg per Kg per Day	Mg per Pound per Day
Histidine	8–12	3.6–5.4
Isoleucine	10	4.5
Leucine	14	6.4
Lysine	12	5.5
Methionine + cystine[b]	13	6.0
Phenylananine	14	6.4
Threonine	7	3.2
Tryptophan	3.5	1.6
Valine	10	4.5

[a] Recommended Daily Allowances, 10th ed., Washington, DC: National Academy Press, 1989, p. 57.
[b] Cystine is a nonessential amino acid that can be ingested or can be made from methionine; thus, the two are often listed together.

nitrogen is found only in protein. Protein is essential for building nearly every part of the body.

There are 4 calories in 1 gram of protein. Adults require 0.75 grams of protein per kilogram of body weight per day. This translates into one-third of a gram of protein per pound. So, an easy estimate for your protein requirements in grams per day would be to divide your body weight by 3. For instance, if you weigh 150 pounds, you need about 50 grams of protein per day.

To make anything in your body, including muscle, you must first have all of the necessary amino acids. Some of them your body can manufacture, while others you must get from your food.

Those amino acids that you must get from your food are called the *essential amino acids,* while the others that you can make are known as the *nonessential amino acids.* During childhood, 9 of the 22 amino acids are essential, while in adulthood we acquire the ability to synthesize one additional amino acid, leaving us with 8 essential amino acids.

Amino acids cannot be stored in the body. Therefore, people need to consume their minimum amounts of protein every day. If adequate protein is not consumed, the body immediately begins to break down tissue (usually beginning with muscle tissue) to release the essential amino acids. If even one essential amino acid is lacking, the other essential ones are not able to work to their capacities. For example, if methionine (the most commonly lacking amino acid) is present at 60 percent of the minimum requirement, the other seven essential amino acids are limited to near 60 percent of their potential. When they are not used, amino acids are excreted in the urine.

Animal products (i.e., fish, poultry, and beef) and animal by-products (i.e., milk, eggs, cheese) are rich in readily usable protein. This means that when you eat animal products or by-products, the protein you consume can be converted into protein in your body because these sources have all of the essential amino acids in them. These foods are called *complete protein sources*.

Incomplete protein sources are any other food sources that provide protein but not all of the essential amino acids. Some examples are beans, peas, and nuts. These food sources must be combined with other food sources that have the missing essential amino acids so that you can make protein in your body. Some examples of complementary foods are rice and beans, and peanut butter on whole-wheat bread.

Fat

Fat is made of carbon, hydrogen and oxygen. There are 9 calories in 1 gram of fat. In the body, fat is used to develop the myelin sheath that surrounds the nerves. It also aids in the absorption of vitamins A, D, E, and K, which are the fat-soluble vitamins. It serves as a protective layer around our vital organs, and it is a great insulator against the cold. It is also a great concentrated energy source. Of course, its most redeeming quality is that it adds flavor and juiciness to food!

Just as protein is broken down into different kinds of nitrogen compounds called amino acids, there are also different kinds of fats (fatty acids): saturated fats, monounsaturated fats, and polyunsaturated fats.

Saturated fats are "saturated" with hydrogen atoms. They are generally solid at room temperature and are most likely found in animal fats, eggs, and whole-milk products. Since these are the fats that are primarily responsible for raising the blood cholesterol level and hardening the arteries, they should be minimized.

Monounsaturated fats (oleic fatty acids) have room for two hydrogen ions to double-bind to one carbon. They are liquid at room temperature and are found in great amounts in olive, peanut, and canola (rapeseed) oils. Dietary monounsaturated fats have been shown to have the greatest effect on the efflux of cholesterol, thereby contributing a positive effect on atherosclerosis.

Polyunsaturated fats (linoleic fatty acids) have at least two carbon double bonds available, which translates into space for at least four hydrogen ions. Poly-unsaturated fats are also liquid at room temperature and are found in the highest proportions in vegetable sources. Safflower, corn, and linseed oils are good sources of this type of fat. Polyunsaturated fatty acids of the omega-3 type may also contribute to the prevention of atherosclerosis.

Trans-fats, often called "partially hardened fats" or "partially hydrogenated," are another type of fat that result from adding hydrogen to poly-unsaturated fats to make them harder, such as when making safflower oil into a margarine. Evidence indicates that these fats may be at least as harmful as the saturated fats. So when you see "partially hydrogenated" on your cookie or cracker packages, those foods are not that good for you.

We eat too much fat. The minimum requirement for fat in the diet is considered to be somewhere between 10 and 20 percent of the total calories consumed. The absolute maximum should be 30 percent, which is the amount now recommended for the American diet. Most of us, however, consume between 35 and 50 percent of our total calories in fats. Also, our typical diet is very high in saturated fats—the type that we want to avoid.

Our high fat intake, most of which is saturated, tends to raise blood cholesterol levels in many people. For those interested in decreasing the chances of developing hardened arteries by lowering their blood cholesterol level, follow a diet low in fat (with the saturated fat intake at 10 percent or less of the total diet) and consume fewer than 300 milligrams of cholesterol daily. Put another way, keep the total calories from fat under a third of your total intake, and eat twice as much poly-unsaturated and monounsaturated fats as saturated fat. Reducing fat also decreases cancer risks.

When buying foods, especially cookies and crackers, always check the type of fat used. Avoid those with palm kernel oil and coconut oil. Also be aware of the hydrogenated oils used. Although a hydrogenated safflower or canola oil may still have an acceptable fat ratio, a hydrogenated peanut or cottonseed oil may not contain the desired levels of unsaturated fats.

Carbohydrates

Carbohydrates are made from carbon, hydrogen, and oxygen, just as are fats, but "carbs" are generally a simpler type of molecule. There are 4 calories in 1 gram of carbohydrate. If not utilized immediately for energy as sugar (glucose), they are either stored in the body as *glycogen* (the stored form of glucose) or synthesized into fat and stored. Some carbohydrates cannot be broken down by the body's digestive processes. These are called *fibers* and will be discussed later. Of the digestible carbohydrates, we will separate them into two categories: simple and complex.

Simple carbohydrates are the most readily usable energy source in the body and include such things as sugar, honey, and fruit. *Complex carbohydrates* are the starches. They also break down into sugar for energy, but their breakdown is slower than with simple carbs. Also, complex carbohydrates bring with them various vitamins and minerals.

People in the United States often eat too many simple carbohydrates—the so-called empty calories. They are empty because they have no vitamins, minerals, or fibers. While a person who uses a great deal of energy can consume these empty calories without potential weight gain, most of us find these empty calories settling on our hips. For example, the average person consumes 125 pounds of sugar per year, which is equivalent to 1 teaspoon every 40 minutes, night and day! Since each teaspoon of sugar contains 17 calories, this amounts to 231,000 calories, or 66 pounds of potential body fat if this energy is not used as fuel for daily living.

High-carbohydrate diets that are especially high in sugar may be hazardous to one's health. They can increase the amount of triglycerides produced in the liver. These triglycerides are blood fats and possible developers of hardened arteries. Also, a diet high in simple carbohydrates can lead to obesity, which can then result in the development of late-onset diabetes.

Fiber

Fiber is that part of the foods we take in that is not digestible. Fiber helps move the food through the intestines by increasing their peristaltic action. Vegetable fibers are made up chiefly of *cellulose,* an indigestible carbohydrate that is the main ingredient in the cell walls of plants. Plant-eating animals, such as cows, can digest cellulose. Meat-eating animals, such as humans, do not have the proper enzymes in their digestive tracts to metabolize cellulose.

Bran (which includes the husks of wheat, oats, rice, rye, and corn) is another type of fiber. It is indigestible because of the silica in the outer husks. Some of the fibers, such as wheat bran, are insoluble. Their major function is to add bulk to the feces and to speed the digested foods through the intestines. This reduces one's risk of constipation, intestinal cancer, appendicitis, and diverticulosis.

Some types of fibers are soluble; that is, they can pick up certain substances such as dietary cholesterol. Pectin, commonly found in raw fruits (especially apple skins), oat and rice brans, and some gums from the seeds and stems of tropical plants (e.g., guar and xanthin) are examples of soluble fibers. These pick up cholesterols as they move through the intestines.

Foods high in fiber are also valuable in weight-reducing diets because they speed the passage of foods through the digestive tract, thereby cutting the amount of possible absorption time. They also cut the amount of hunger experienced by a dieter because they fill the stomach. A larger salad with a diet dressing might give the person very few calories but still enough cellulose to fill the stomach, cut the hunger, and move other foods through the intestinal passage.

Food processing often removes the natural fiber from the food. This is one of the primary reasons that we, in the Western world, have relatively low amounts of fiber in our diet. For instance, white bread has only a trace of fiber—about 9 grams in a loaf— while old-fashioned whole-wheat bread has 70 grams. Also, when you peel a carrot or an apple, you remove much of the fiber.

Dietitians urge that people include more fiber in their diets, particularly whole-grain cereals, bran, and fibrous vegetables. Root vegetables (carrots, beets and turnips) and leafy vegetables are very good sources of fiber. The average American diet has between 10 and 20 grams of fiber in it per day. We also have about twice the rate of colon cancer in this country versus other countries whose citizens eat more fiber. This is why the National Cancer Institute has recommended that we consume between 25 and 35 grams of fiber per day.

Vitamins

Vitamins are organic compounds that are essential in small amounts for the growth and development of animals and humans. They act as enzymes (catalysts) that facilitate many of the body processes to occur. Although great controversy surrounds the importance of consuming excess vitamins, it is acknowledged that we need a minimum amount of vitamins for proper functioning.

Some vitamins are soluble only in water; others need fat to be absorbed by the body. The water-soluble vitamins, B complex and C, are more fragile than the fat-soluble vitamins. This is because they are more easily destroyed by the heat of cooking, and if boiled, they lose some of their potency into the water.

The fat-soluble vitamins, A, D, E, and K, need oils in the intestines to be absorbed by the body. They are more stable than the water-soluble vitamins and are not destroyed by normal cooking methods. Because they are stored in the body, there is the possibility of ingesting too much of them, especially vitamins A and D.

Nutritional researchers disagree as to whether vitamin supplements are necessary; however, more are seeing the necessity for supplementation with the vitamins that neutralize the free oxygen radicals. *Free oxygen radicals* are harmful substances produced by many natural body processes, air pollution and smoke. Physical exercise, for all of its benefits, is one producer of free oxygen radicals. Supplementation with antioxidants (beta carotene, vitamins C and E) reduces the free oxygen radicals that seem to be responsible for some cancers and other diseases. Dr. Ken Cooper, the man who coined the term *aerobics* and developed the first world-recognized fitness program, suggests a minimum supplementation of 400 IU of vitamin E, 1,000 milli-grams of vitamin C, and 25,000 milligrams of beta carotene daily to counteract the potential damage done to the body by free oxygen radicals.

Minerals

Minerals are usually structural components of the body, but they sometimes participate in certain body processes. The body uses many minerals—phosphorus, calcium, and magnesium for strong teeth and bones; zinc for growth; chromium for carbo-hydrate metabolism; and copper and iron for hemoglobin produc-tion in the blood.

Iron is used primarily in devel-oping hemoglobin, which carries the oxygen in the red blood cells. Women need more iron than men until they go through menopause (18 milligrams a day), at which time their iron requirements drop to that of men (10 milligrams a day). Iron deficiency, common in women athletes, may impair athletic performance and should be corrected with supplementation.

Magnesium is the eighth most abundant element on the Earth's surface. It seems to help activate enzymes essential to energy transfer. It is crucial for effective contraction of the muscles. Exercise depletes this element so supplementation may be called for. When it is not present in sufficient amounts, twitching, tremors, and undue anxiety may develop.

Calcium is primarily responsible for the building of strong bones and teeth. For this reason, it seems obvious that a diet that is chronically low in calcium would have a negative effect on one's bone strength. The result of this is brittle and porous bones as one gets older, a condition known as *osteoporosis*. The inclusion of adequate calcium (which may be higher than the current RDA—Recommended Daily Allowance) in teenage and young adult years can aid in the development of peak bone mass, which can help prevent osteoporosis later on in life. Calcium is also necessary for strong teeth, nerve transmissions, blood clotting, and muscle contractions. Without enough calcium, muscle cramps often result. Skipping milk with its necessary calcium may be the cause of menstrual cramping for some girls. The uterus is a muscle, and muscles need both sodium and calcium for proper contractile functioning.

Phytochemicals

Phytochemicals (*phyto* is Greek for "plant") include thousands of chemical compounds that are found in plants. Some of these are vitamins and many have no known effect on us; however, more and more are being found to be highly beneficial.

In the past, the phytonutrients found in fruits and vegetables were classified as vitamins: flavonoids were known as vitamin P, cabbage factors (glucosinolates and indoles) were called vitamin U, and ubiquinone was vitamin Q. Tocopherol somehow stayed on the list as vitamin E. Vitamin designation was dropped for the other nutrients because specific deficiency symptoms could not be established. *Vita* means "life," so if the compound could not be found to be absolutely essential for life, it was dropped as a "vitamin" but is now classified as a phytochemical.

Various phytochemicals have been found to reduce the chance of cancers developing, lower the risk of heart attack, decrease blood pressure, and increase immunity factors. Few of these have been reduced to pill form, such as vitamin pills, so they must be consumed in fruits and vegetables daily. It is suggested that each of us consume at least five servings of raw fruits or vegetables daily. Since many of the phytochemicals are heat-sensitive, cooking can destroy some or all of the active ingredients.

Endurance and Strength Training

Fatigue is often a factor in losing the last few points of a game or in incurring an injury. As players get tired, they make more physical errors, leading to injury. Being in shape for badminton can help avoid these pitfalls and increase your enjoyment from playing the game.

Increasing the capacity of your *cardiovascular system* (heart, lungs, and arteries) is essential to enable you to supply oxygen to all of the muscles in the body for a period of time long enough to maintain the pace of an extended game or an all-day tournament.

Developing muscular endurance is also important. The muscles that are used continually during a match must have the ability to absorb oxygen and other fuels so that they do not tire. The legs (calf and thigh muscles) and the hitting arm (triceps, rotator cuff and upper chest muscles) are most subject to fatigue. They must therefore be exercised for endurance.

Overload Principle

The main factor in improving fitness of any kind is the overload principle. *Overload* means to push yourself each time to do a little more than you are accustomed to doing. Without this factor there will be no improvement.

There are three ways to overload: intensity, duration, and frequency:

Intensity: how hard you do something

Duration: how long you do something

Frequency: how often you do something

The intensity of exercise may be measured by monitoring your pulse rate, either during or immediately following exercise. The higher the pulse rate, the harder the heart is working. The same task should become easier as your condition improves, thereby enabling you to work at higher intensities; such as all-out play for a longer period of time.

Duration is measured by how long a period of time you continue to exercise—playing for longer periods of time each time you play, gradually conditioning the heart to work a little longer without rest.

Frequency is measured by how often or how many times a week you play, run, or lift weights. Running four times per week instead of three times is an increase in frequency.

To improve the cardiovascular system, you must overload one or more of these principles of fitness. The safest and easiest on the body to overload is frequency. This may be done by playing more times per week at the same intensity.

Aerobic Training

The *cardiorespiratory system* (heart, arteries, and lungs) can be improved through the performance of exercises that elevate the pulse rate for an extended period of time. These activities, known as *aerobic exercises,* increase the body's ability to supply oxygen to the cells.

To contract (shorten), muscle cells need fuel, which they receive from blood cells in the form of nutrients. The nutrients are metabolized from the food we eat. Oxygen is a necessity in order for the cells to utilize these nutrients. When the heart and lungs cannot supply oxygen at a rate fast enough to keep up with the demands placed on it by the body (a phenomenon known as *oxygen debt*), fatigue sets in and efficiency decreases.

Aerobic exercises train or condition the body to adapt to this demand by strengthening the mechanisms involved: the heart, lungs, and arteries. They do this by forcing the heart to work much harder than normal for 20 to 30 minutes.

The bottom line is that exercising aerobically increases maximal oxygen consumption by improving the efficiency of supply and delivery. You may select any activity that maintains your pulse in the target pulse zone (described later) for an extended period of time. The most commonly recommended activities are running, jogging, cycling, stationary running, rope jumping, walking, and swimming.

All of those activities elevate the pulse rate to a level high enough to attain a training effect, but not so high as to cause fatigue or the need for a rest. The individual should be able to continue the exercise for a length of time—long enough to attain a training effect.

Target Pulse Rate

One way to ensure you are exercising aerobically is to monitor your pulse rate to keep it in the *target pulse zone,* the pulse level the body should maintain to reap the benefits of aerobic training. To determine your target pulse zone, first find your maximum exercise pulse by subtracting your age from 220. Your target pulse zone is between 65 and 90 percent of your maximum exercise pulse. If the exercise is too intense, the pulse will rise above the upper limit of your target pulse zone, and breathing will become more difficult as a result of the body's attempt to keep up with this extreme oxygen demand. Consider this example:

$220 - 20$ years old $= 200$ (your maximum projected heart rate)

200×90 percent $(0.9) = 180$ heart rate a 90 percent level for a 20-year-old

200×65 percent $(0.65) = 130$ heart rate a 65 percent level for a 20-year-old.

This 20-year-old person should maintain a pulse rate of 130 to 160 for 20 to 30 minutes for the body to receive the benefits of aerobic training. This should be done a minimum of three or four times each week. (See the box for the more complicated Karvonen formula that is more generally used today.)

The Karvonen Formula

Scientists are continuing to improve their knowledge of how best our bodies can work. The Finnish scientist Karvonen has improved on the simple formula of "220 minus your age" as the maximum heart rate. He starts with that number but then subtracts the resting pulse rate to determine the "heart rate reserve."

1. First take 220 minus your age. This is your maximum heart rate (MHR).

2. Next you will need to determine your resting pulse rate (Rest HR). Take this while lying in bed in the morning before you get up. Use your index and middle fingers and locate your pulse either on the side of your neck (carotid artery) or on the wrist just above the thumb. Count the number of pulse beats in a minute, or take your pulse for 15 seconds and multiply by 4 to determine the total for a minute.

3. Subtract the resting pulse rate from the maximum pulse rate.

   MHR − Rest HR = heart rate reserve (HRR)

4. Now you will determine your maximum and minimum pulse rates for an effective work out. For the average person, the high end will be the heart rate reserve multiplied by 80 percent (0.80), then added to the resting pulse rate:

   HRR × 0.80) + Rest HR = maximum desirable heart rate during exercise

5. Next find the minimal acceptable level for your work out by taking the heart rate reserve (HRR), multiplying it by 60 percent (0.60), and then adding in your resting pulse rate.

   (HRR × 0.60) + Rest HR = minimum desirable heart rate during exercise

These two percentages (60 and 80 percent) are not set in stone. If you had medical problems or were in very poor condition, you might use a number between 40 percent and 55 percent to set your minimal pulse rate. If you were very fit or a competitive athlete, you might use 85 or 90 percent to set your high-end exercise pulse rate.

Let's use an example of how a 20-year-old would determine the target training pulse range. Assume that her resting pulse rate was 70.

Minimum target heart rate (220 − 20 = 200 + 70 = 270) × 0.60 = 162

Maximum target heart rate (220 − 20 = 200 + 70 = 270) × 0.80 = 216

For a 40-year-old with a resting pulse of 65, the target heart rates would be

Minimum target heart rate (220 − 40 = 180 + 65 = 245) × 0.60 = 147

Maximum target heart rate (220 − 40 = 180 + 65 = 245) × 0.80 = 196

Strength Training

Badminton players may not realize how much strength they need for the game. The quick starts and the jumping ability needed to play a game are based on your body's ability to use its strength quickly.

A Specific Strength Program for Badminton

While an overall body building program may be good for everyone, special exercises can be particularly beneficial to badminton players. Abdominal and lower-back strength are useful in nearly every sport. Badminton players should strengthen their shoulders, arms, and wrists as well as their leg muscles. If you belong to a gym, you can do the following exercises with barbells or dumbbells. However, we will illustrate them with other types of resistance —books, a partner or a broom.

Abdominal strength is important for everyone. Sufficient strength helps keep our abdomens tucked in for better posture. In fact, the abdominals, along with the lower back, are the two most important areas for strength in our bodies. In athletics the abdominals help stabilize the pelvis, so they are essential in every action that involves the hip joints—running, jumping, and the hip rotation in a hard overhead or smash.

Lie on your back. To attempt to isolate your abdominals, you should bend your knees as much as possible so that the muscles that flex the hip joint (bringing the thighs forward and upward) will not work as much. You should also keep your hips (your belt) on the mat when doing an abdominal exercise. Whenever your hips are pulled off the mat or bench, your hip flexors are working. This is particularly harmful for girls and women who generally have an excessive curvature in their lower backs. (This curvature places a higher pressure on the outside of the disks in the lumbar [lower-back] region. It causes many problems as the person grows older.)

The reason that some hip flexion exercises can increase the curvature of the spine is that some muscles deep inside the pelvis attach from the lower-back bones to the thigh bone. As they get stronger, they pull in on the lower spine and increase the curvature. You will often see this extreme lower-back curve (technically called *lordosis*) in female gymnasts.

Now curl your shoulders forward until your hips are about to leave the floor. Usually you will be able to touch your elbows to your thighs.

Some people aren't sufficiently strong to do this exercise correctly the first time. If this is true for you,

do the exercise this way: Grab the back of your thighs with your hands and pull yourself up to the proper position. When this becomes easy, use only one hand on one thigh to help you curl up. Soon you will be able to do the exercise without using your hands to assist you. The exercise is easier with your hands on your hips and harder with your hands on your chest.

To emphasize the twisting action of a badminton shot, twist your torso as you rise up. First the left shoulder toward the right knee, then the right shoulder toward the left knee.

Lower-back exercises are probably the most important for the average person to do because lower-back injuries, especially muscle pulls, are so common. The lower-back muscles are particularly important in badminton because of the quick bending movements involved. And, of course, they are essential in maintaining good posture because they are the muscles that hold our chests up by lifting our rib cages. They pull the back of the rib cage down. This raises the front of the rib cage and our chests come with our ribs.

Back arches can be done on the floor. Just lie face down and raise your shoulders and knees slightly off the floor. You do not want a big arch because hyperextending the backbone is not a safe exercise. You can also do this exercise twisting, lifting the right shoulder higher on one arch then the left shoulder higher on the next.

In a gym there may be a "Roman chair" available; if so,

using one increases the resistance you can gain in your exercise. In a Roman chair you will put your hips on the small saddle, hook your feet under a bar, bend forward at the waist about 30 degrees, and then straighten your back, being careful not to hyperextend.

Wrist strength is critical to effective badminton play. No sport requires the wrist quickness of badminton. The wrist flexors are used in the forehand actions. Grab a broom with your palm facing upward and the handle of the broom held in a nearly straight line with the lower part of the arm. Allow the weight of the broom to extend your wrist backward as far as possible, and then flex your wrist upward as far as it will go. Only the wrist should move. If you are not too strong, hold the broom handle closer to the middle. If you are quite strong, hold it at the end. You can also do this exercise using your own hand as the resistance. Use one hand to resist the other and perform the same action as with the broom. You can also use a badminton racket with a partner giving resistance to the end of the racket.

If you are at a gym, sit down while straddling a bench. With a barbell in your hands, with your palms up and the back of your forearms on the bench, let the weight hyperextend your wrist and then flex your wrist forward. This exercise can also be done with a dumbbell exercising one wrist then the other.

An exercise that will assist in developing wrist strength and also develop strength in the fingers is the tennis ball squeeze. Simply find an old soft tennis ball and squeeze it.

Wrist *pronation* (turning the lower arm inward) also occurs in most forehand shots in which the wrist is flexing. To strengthen this muscle action, grab the broom handle with your thumb facing away from the midline of your body and so that the broom handle is held perpendicular to your arm. The heavier end of the broom should be on the thumb side of your hand and dropped downward. Turn your lower arm so that the heavy end of the broom moves upward. When it is straight up, this completes the pronation part of the exercise.

For your backhand shots, you will want a *supination* action (turning your lower arm outward). To strengthen this action, let the heavy end of the broom continue moving past the vertical and inward until the heavy end is closer to the midline of your body and is as low as it will drop. The supination action begins as you lift the heavy end of the broom upwards to the vertical. Continue this rotary action of the broom until your arm is tired. To increase the resistance and gain more strength, have a partner give some resistance to the end of the broom as it is moving upward.

The *back of the wrists* (wrist extensors) are important in all of your backhand shots. Using the broom with the heavy end extended in a line with your arm and your palm facing downward, lift the broom upward using only your wrist.

If you are in a gym, while sitting and straddling a bench and your hands grasping the barbell (palms down), let the barbell flex your wrists then extend your wrists upward. This exercise will strengthen the back of your forearms. You will probably be able to use only about two-thirds of the weight that you were able to do in the wrist flexion exercise.

The *rotator cuff muscles* turn the upper arm in the shoulder socket. These very important muscles come into play in most badminton shots. Because these muscles are quite small, they are often injured. They should therefore be exercised for both maximum strength and for injury prevention.

Using the same broom, gripped so that it is held perpendicular to your arm, and the arm extended at shoulder height and directly to the side of the body, rotate the broom so that the heavy end of the broom moves in a circular path around your hand. Only the upper arm rotates in the shoulder socket.

If at a gym, while lying on your back on a bench holding a dumbbell, with your elbow at a 90-degree angle to your side, bring the dumbbell to a vertical position and then continue the action until the weight is touching your abdomen. Return to the starting position. This exercise will work two different actions of the rotator cuff muscles.

Hip abduction and adduction exercises are important because of the quick lateral movements required in badminton. *Abduction* is the name for the movement in which the thigh moves in a lateral plane to the side; *adduction* is the action of the thigh moving to the original position. If you were doing jumping jacks, your legs would be abducting and adducting with each complete movement.

With a partner, you lie on your back with your partner kneeling at your feet, holding the outside of your feet or lower legs and giving resistance. Push your legs apart (abduction) as far as they will go with your partner resisting. Then the partner changes the resistance to the inside of your ankles and you bring your legs back together. At a gym, use the abduction and adduction machines.

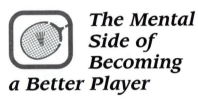 ## The Mental Side of Becoming a Better Player

Wishing won't make you a better player. You must practice learning the physical skills of badminton. This practice will take place primarily on the court. While it is important to work out physically to condition your body, you can also learn to become a better player at home by practicing mentally. Championship athletes have known for years that mental practice can help performance. Only recently have sports psychologists refined methods of utilizing the mind's contribution to the game.

Mental imagery, or visualization, is the name given to this type of mental practice. It can be done externally, observing good players in person or on a videotape, or internally, imagining watching yourself from outside your body. While mentally experiencing your game, you can practice your shots and footwork or even strategy and court positioning. You can practice whatever aspect of your game you would like to improve. If your service return is a problem, imagine yourself ready for the return. The imaginary opponent serves to your left. Feel yourself

Checklist for Mental Imagery

1. Do you watch top-level badminton players or videotapes of badminton skills?

2. Have you tried being the star in your own mental movie by closing your eyes and performing skills to perfection?

3. Do you always see yourself completing all aspects of the skill perfectly and include a successful finish?

4. Do you practice all aspects of the game mentally?

5. Are you always positive in your instructions to yourself?

making the proper play. Move toward the shuttlecock, get your racket in proper position, watch the shuttle, and make the perfect shot. Think of keeping your head down and eyes focused on the shuttle.

Concentration is another major area of mental practice. You must have a specific focus to play at your maximum potential. That point of focus will vary during a rally. Failure to focus on the shuttle all the way to the point of contact and while it is on your racket is probably the most common and critical error at every level of badminton. Slow-motion studies reveal that most people take their eyes off of the shuttle when it is still 4 to 6 feet away from them. They look at where they want to hit instead of concentrating on the point of contact of the shuttle and the racket.

Summary

Nutrition

1. In our lives, as well as on the badminton court, we will profit from better nutrition and more effective aerobic conditioning.

2. The basic macronutrients are protein, fat, carbohydrate. Water is also essential.

3. Proteins are made of amino acids. Eight of these are considered to be essential and should be consumed daily.

4. Our bodies need fats, about 10 to 20 percent of our daily caloric intake.

5. Saturated fats and cholesterol are often risk factors for heart disease.

6. The greatest percentage of our diets should be in complex carbohydrates, those containing vitamins, minerals, and fiber.

7. While proteins, fats, and carbohydrates (macronutrients) are the largest amount of nutrients consumed, vitamins, minerals and phytochemicals (micronutrients) are also essential.

8. Vitamins help body processes to happen. They break down the macronutrients and accomplish other essential body functions.

9. Free oxygen radicals are harmful byproducts of living which can be reduced by some vitamins (beta carotene, vitamins C and E).

10. Minerals are necessary building blocks of the body and are essential in every tissue.

11. Phytochemicals are desirable, possibly necessary, elements found in plants that may aid us in obtaining a higher level of nutrition.

12. Vitamin supplementation may be necessary for many people. Most will apparently profit from antioxidant supplementation.

Endurance and Strength Training

1. Conditioning can provide the means for the player to be able to maintain a high skill level throughout the entire game and avoid errors and injuries that may be attributed to fatigue.

2. Training is specific. To get into shape to play badminton, you must play and practice the game.

3. High-level badminton demands improvement of the cardiovascular system and strengthening of the muscles.

4. For best results, the overload principle should provide the basis for your fitness program.

5. There are three ways to overload: intensity, duration, and frequency.

6. Aerobic training can improve the efficiency of the cardio-vascular system.

7. Aerobic training results in the phenomenon known as a *training effect*.

8. Anaerobic exercises are activities of higher intensity and lower duration, while aerobic exercises are activities of lower intensity and higher duration.

9. To benefit from the results of aerobic training, the pulse must remain in the target pulse zone all during the activity.

10. The badminton player should exercise the specific muscular actions that are specially designed to improve success in this sport.

The Mental Side of Becoming a Better Player

1. The complete badminton player must make use of his or her maximum mental potentials. There are various ways to improve one's badminton off the court:

   a. Imagery—in which a person visualizes the techniques and the game situations which may be encountered

   b. Concentration—in which the player focuses on the shuttle all the way to the point of contact

Appendix
*Laws of Badminton**

Laws

1. **COURT**

   1.1 The court shall be a rectangle and laid out as in the following Diagram "A" (except in the case provided for in Law 1.5) and to the measurements there shown, defined by lines 40 mm wide.

   1.2 The lines shall be easily distinguishable and preferably be colored white or yellow.

   1.3.1 To show the zone in which a shuttle of correct pace lands when tested (Law 4.4), an additional four marks 40 mm by 40 mm may be made inside each side line for singles of the right service court, 530 mm and 990 mm from the back boundary line.

   1.3.2 In making these marks, their width shall be within the measurement given, *i.e.*, the marks will be from 530 mm to 570 mm and from 950 mm to 990 mm from the outside of the back boundary line.

   1.4 All lines form part of the area which they define.

   1.5 Where space does not permit the marking out of a court for doubles, a court may be marked out for singles only as in Diagram "B." The back boundary lines become also the long service lines, and the posts or the strips of material representing them (Law 2.2), shall be placed on the side lines.

2. **POSTS**

   2.1 The posts shall be 1.55 meters in height from the surface of the court. They shall be sufficiently firm to remain vertical and keep the net strained as provided in Law 3, and shall be placed on the doubles side lines as shown in Diagram "A".

   2.2 Where it is not practicable to have posts on the side lines, some method must be used to indicate the position of the sidelines where they pass under the net, e.g., by the use of thin posts or strips of material 40 mm wide, fixed to the side lines and rising vertically to the net cord.

   2.3 On a court marked for doubles, the posts or strips of material representing the posts shall be placed on the side lines for doubles, irrespective of whether singles or doubles is being played.

3. **NET**

   3.1 The net shall be made of fine cord of dark color and even thickness with a mesh not less than 15 mm and not more than 20 mm.

   3.2 The net shall be 760 mm (2 ft. 6 inches) in depth.

   3.3 The top of the net shall be edged with a 75 mm (3 inch) white tape doubled over a cord or cable running through the tape. This tape must rest upon the cord or cable.

   3.4 The cord or cable shall be of sufficient size and weight to be firmly stretched flush with the top of the posts.

   3.5 The top of the net from the surface of the court shall be 1.524 meters (5 feet) at the center of the court and 1.55 meters (5 feet 1 inch) over the side lines for doubles.

---

* Excerpted and reprinted from *Official Rules of Play*, pps. 21–49, with permission from the United States Badminton Association.

Diagram A

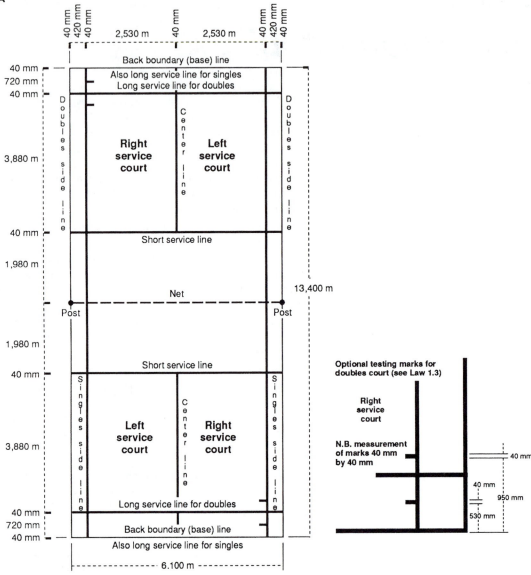

Note: Court can be used for both singles and doubles play.

Diagonal length of full court = 14.723 m

**Optional testing marks shown opposite.

3.6 There shall be no gaps between the ends of the net and the posts. If necessary, the full depth of the net should be tied at the ends.

4. SHUTTLE

Principles

The shuttle may be made from natural and/or synthetic materials. Whatever material the shuttle is made from, the flight characteristics, generally, should be similar to those produced by a natural feathered shuttle with a cork base covered by a thin layer of leather.

Having regard to the Principles:

4.1 *General Design*

4.1.1 The shuttle shall have 16 feathers fixed in the base.

Diagram B

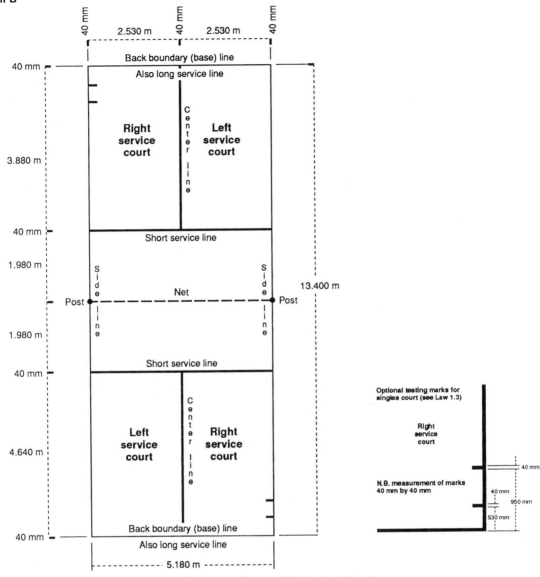

Note: Court can be used for singles play only.

Diagonal length of singles court = 14.366 m

**Optional testing marks shown opposite

4.1.2 The feathers can have a variable length from 64 mm to 70 mm, but in each shuttle they shall be the same length when measured from the tip to the top of the base.

4.1.3 The tips of the feathers shall form a circle with a diameter from 58 mm to 68 mm.

4.1.4 The feathers shall be fastened firmly with thread or other suitable material.

4.1.5 The base shall be:

- 25 mm to 28 mm in diameter
- rounded on the bottom

4.2 *Weight*

The shuttle shall weigh from 4.74 to 5.50 grams.

4.3 *Non-Feathered Shuttle*

4.3.1 The skirt, or simulation of feathers in synthetic materials, replaces natural feathers.

4.3.2 The base is described in Law 4.1.5.

4.3.3 Measurements and weight shall be as in Laws 4.1.2, 4.1.3 and 4.2. However, because of the difference of the specific gravity and behavior of synthetic materials in comparison with feathers, a variation of up to ten percent is acceptable.

4.4 *Shuttle Testing*

4.4.1 To test a shuttle, use a full underhand stroke which makes contact with the shuttle over the back boundary line. The shuttle shall be hit at an upward angle and in a direction parallel to the side lines.

4.4.2 A shuttle of correct pace will land not less than 530 mm and not more than 990 mm short of the other back boundary line.

4.5 *Modifications*

Subject to there being no variation in the general design, pace and flight of the shuttle, modifications in the above specifications may be made with the approval of the National Organization concerned:

4.5.1 in places where atmospheric conditions due to either altitude or climate make the standard shuttle unsuitable; or

4.5.2 if special circumstances exist which make it otherwise necessary in the interests of the game.

5. RACKET

5.1 The hitting surface of the racket shall be flat and consist of a pattern of crossed strings connected to a frame and either alternately interlaced or bonded where they cross. The stringing pattern shall be generally uniform and, in particular, not less dense in the center than in any other area.

5.2 The frame of the racket, including the handle, shall not exceed 680 mm in overall length and 230 mm in overall width.

5.3 The overall length of the head shall not exceed 290 mm.

5.4 The strung surface shall not exceed 280 mm in overall length and 220 mm in overall width.

5.5 The racket:

5.5.1 shall be free of attached objects and protrusions, other than those utilized solely and specifically to limit or prevent wear and tear, or vibration, or to distribute weight, or to secure the handle by cord to the player's hand, and which are reasonable in size and placement for such purposes; and

5.5.2 shall be free of any device which makes it possible for a player to change materially the shape of the racket.

6. APPROVED EQUIPMENT

The International Badminton Federation shall rule on any question of whether any racket, shuttle or equipment or any prototypes used in the playing of Badminton complies with the specifications or is otherwise approved or not approved for play. Such ruling may be undertaken on the Federation's initiative or upon application by any party with a bona fide interest therein including any player, equipment manufacturer or National Organization or member thereof.

7. PLAYERS

7.1 "Player" applies to all those taking part in a match.

7.2 The game shall be played, in the case of doubles, by two players a side, or in the case of singles, by one player a side.

7.3 The side having the right to serve shall be called the serving side, and the opposing side shall be called the receiving side.

8. TOSS

8.1 Before commencing play, the opposing sides shall toss and the side winning the toss shall exercise the choice in either or Law 8.1.1 or Law 8.1.2.

    8.1.1 To serve or receive first.

    8.1.2 To start play at one end of the court or the other.

8.2 The side losing the toss shall then exercise the remaining choice.

9. SCORING

9.1 The opposing sides shall play the best of three games unless otherwise arranged. It is permissible to play one game of 21 points by prior arrangement.

9.2 Only the serving side can add a point to its score.

9.3 In doubles and Men's singles a game is won by the first side to score 15 points (21 points in a match consisting of a single game).

9.4 In Women's singles a game is won by the first side to score 11 points, except as provided in Law 9.6.

9.5.1 If the score becomes 13 all or 14 all (9 all or 10 all in Women's singles), (19 or 20 in a 21 point game), the side which first scored 13 or 14 (9 or 10) (19 or 21) shall have the choice of "setting" or "not setting" the game (Law 9.6).

9.5.2 This choice can only be made when the score is first reached and must be made before the next service is delivered.

9.5.3 The relevant side (Law, 9.5.1) is given the opportunity to set at 14 all (10 all in Women's singles) (20 all in a 21 point game) despite any previous decision not to set by that side or the opposite side at 13 all (9 all in Women's singles) (19 all in a 21 point game).

9.6 If the game has been set, the score is called "Love All" and the side first scoring the set number of points (Law 9.6.12 to 9.6.4) wins the game.

    9.6.1 13 all setting to 5 points

    9.6.2 14 all setting to 3 points

    9.6.3 9 all setting to 3 points

    9.6.4 10 all setting to 2 points

    9.6.5 19 all setting to 5 points

    9.6.6 20 all setting to 3 points

9.7 The side winning a game serves first in the next game.

10. CHANGE OF ENDS

10.1 Players shall change ends:

    10.1.1 at the end of the first game;

    10.1.2 prior to the beginning of the third game (if any); and

    10.1.3 in the third game, or in a one game match, when the leading score reaches:

        - 6 in a game of 11 points

        - 8 in a game of 15 points

        - 11 in a game of 21 points

10.2 When players omit to change ends as indicated by Law 10.1, they shall do so immediately the mistake is discovered and the existing score shall stand.

11. SERVICE

11.1 In a correct service:

    11.1.1 neither side shall cause undue delay to the delivery of the service;

    11.1.2 the server and receiver shall stand within diagonally opposite service courts without touching the boundary lines of these service courts; some part of both feet of the server and receiver must remain in contact with the surface of the court in a stationary position until the service is delivered (Law 11.4);

11.1.3 the server's racket shall initially hit the base of the shuttle while the whole of the shuttle is below the server's waist;

11.1.4 the shaft of the server's racket at the instant of hitting the shuttle shall be pointing in a downward direction to such an extent that the whole of the head of the racket is discernably below the whole of the server's hand holding the racket;

11.1.5 the movement of the server's racket must continue forwards after the start of the service (Law 11.2) until the service is delivered; and

11.1.6 the flight of the shuttle shall be upwards from the server's racket to pass over the net, so that, if not intercepted, it falls in the receiver's service court.

11.2 Once the players have taken their positions, the first forward movement of the server's racket is the start of the service.

11.3 The server shall not serve before the receiver is ready, but the receiver shall be considered to have been ready if a return of service is attempted.

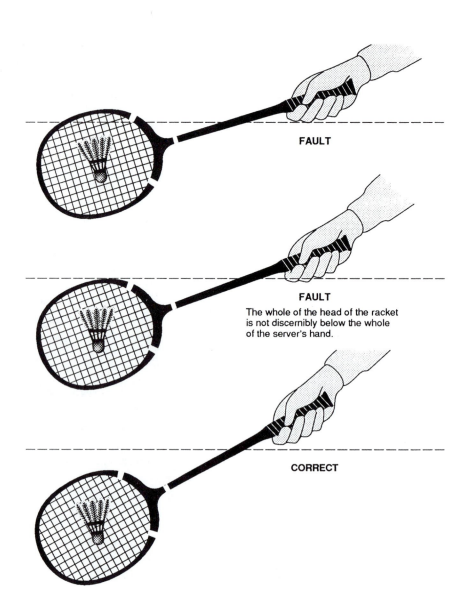

FAULT

FAULT

The whole of the head of the racket is not discernibly below the whole of the server's hand.

CORRECT

11.4   The service is delivered when, once started (Law 11.2), the shuttle is hit by the server's racket or the shuttle lands on the floor.

11.5   In doubles, the partners, may take up any positions which do not unsight the opposing server or receiver.

12. SINGLES

12.1   The players shall serve from, and receive in, their respective right service courts when the server has not scored or has scored an even number of points in that game.

12.2   The players shall serve from, and receive in, their respective left service courts when the server has scored an odd number of points in that game.

12.3   If a game is set, the total points scored by the server in that game shall be used to apply Laws 12.1 and 12.2.

12.4   The shuttle is hit alternately by the server and the receiver until a "fault" is made or the shuttle ceases to be in play.

12.5.1 If the receiver makes a "fault" or the shuttle ceases to be in play because it touches the surface of the court inside the receiver's court, the server scores a point. The server then serves again from the alternate service court.

12.5.2 If the server makes a "fault" or the shuttle ceases to be in play because it touches the surface of the court inside the server's court, the server loses the right to continue serving, and the receiver then becomes the server, with no point scored by either player.

13. DOUBLES

13.1   At the start of a game, and each time a side gains the right to serve, the service shall be delivered from the right service court.

13.2   Only the receiver shall return the service: should the shuttle touch or be hit by the receiver's partner, the serving side scores a point.

13.3.1 After the service is returned, the shuttle is hit by either player of the serving side and then by either player of the receiving side, and so on, until the shuttle ceases to be in play.

13.3.2 After the service is returned, a player may hit the shuttle from any position on that player's side of the net.

13.4.1 If the receiving side makes a "fault" or the shuttle ceases to be in play because it touches the surface of the court inside the receiving side's court, the serving side scores a point, and the server serves again.

13.4.2 If the serving side makes a "fault" or the shuttle ceases to play because it touches the surface of the court inside the serving side's court, the server loses the right to continue serving, with no point scored by either side.

13.5.1 The player who serves at the start of any game shall serve from or receive in, the right service court when that player's side has not scored or has scored an even number of points in that game, and the left service court otherwise.

13.5.2 The player who receives at the start of any game shall receive in, or serve from, the right service court when that player's side has not scored or has scored an even number of points in that game, and the left service court otherwise.

13.5.3 The reverse pattern applies to the partners.

13.5.4 If a game is set, the total points scored by a side in that game shall be used to apply Laws 13.5.1 to 13.5.3.

13.6   Service in any turn of serving shall be delivered from alternate service courts, except as provided in Laws 14 and 16.

13.7   The right to serve passes consecutively from the initial server in any game to the initial receiver in that game, and then consecutively from that player to that player's partner and then to one of the opponents and then the opponent's partner, and so on.

13.8   No player shall serve out of turn, receive out of turn, or receive two consecutive services in the same game, except as provided in Laws 14 and 16.

13.9 Either player of the winning side may serve first in the next game and either player of the losing side may receive.

14. SERVICE COURT ERRORS

14.1 A service court error has been made when a player:

14.1.1 has served out of turn;

14.1.2 has served from the wrong service court; or

14.1.3 standing in the wrong service court, was prepared to receive the service and it has been delivered.

14.2 When a service court error has been made, then

14.2.1 if the error is discovered before the next service is delivered, it is a "let" unless only one side was at fault and lost the rally, in which case the error shall not be corrected.

14.2.2 if the error is not discovered before the next service is delivered, the error shall not be corrected.

14.3 If there is a "let" because of a service court error, the rally is replayed with the error corrected.

14.4 If a service court error is not to be corrected, play in that game shall proceed without changing the players' new service courts (nor, when relevant, the new order of serving).

15. FAULTS

It is a "fault":

15.1 if a service is not correct (Law 11.1);

15.2 if the server, in attempting to serve, misses the shuttle;

15.3 if after passing over the net on service, the shuttle is caught in or on the net;

15.4 if in play, the shuttle;

15.4.1 lands outside the boundaries of the court;

15.4.2 passes through or under the net;

15.4.3 fails to pass the net;

15.4.4 touches the roof, ceiling, or side walls;

15.4.5 touches the person or dress of a player; or

15.4.6 touches any other object or person outside the immediate surroundings of the court;

(Where necessary on account of the structure of the building, the local badminton authority may, subject to the right of veto of its National Organization, make bye–laws dealing with cases in which a shuttle touches an obstruction).

15.5 if, when in play, the initial point of contact with the shuttle is not on the striker's side of the net. (The striker may, however, follow the shuttle over the net with the racket in the course of a stroke).

15.6 if, when the shuttle is in play, a player:

15.6.1 touches the net or its supports with racket, person or dress

15.6.2 Invades an opponent's court *over the net* with racket or person except as permitted in Law 15.5;

15.6.3 Invades an opponent's court *under the net* with racket or person such that an opponent is obstructed or distracted; or

15.6.4 Obstructs an opponent, *i.e.* prevents an opponent from making a legal stroke where the shuttle is followed over the net;

15.7 if, in play, a player deliberately distracts an opponent by any action such as shouting or making gestures;

15.8   if, in play, the shuttle;

    15.8.1   be caught and held on the racket and then slung during the execution of a stroke;

    15.8.2   be hit twice in succession by the same player with two strokes; (a double hit by one player with one stroke is not a fault) or

    15.8.3   be hit by a player and the player's partner successively;

    15.8.4   Touches a player's racket and continues toward the back of that player's court.

15.9   if a player is guilty of flagrant, repeated or persistent offenses under Law 18.

16. LETS

"Let" is called by the Umpire, or by a player (if there is not Umpire) to halt play.

16.1   A "let" may be given for any unforeseen or accidental occurrence.

16.2   If a shuttle, after passing over the net, is caught in or on the net, it is a "let" except during service.

16.3   If during service, the receiver and server are both faulted at the same time, it shall be a "let."

16.4   If the server serves before the receiver is ready it shall be a "let."

16.5   If during play, the shuttle disintegrates and the base completely separates from the rest of the shuttle, it shall be a "let."

16.6   If a Line Judge is unsighted and the Umpire is unable to make a decision, it shall be a "let."

16.7   When a "let" occurs, the play since the last service shall not count, and the player who served shall serve again, except when Law 14 is applicable.

17. SHUTTLE NOT IN PLAY

A shuttle is not in play when:

17.1   it strikes the net and remains attached there or suspended on top;

17.2   it strikes the net or post and starts to fall towards the surface of the court on the striker's side of the net;

17.3   it hits the surface of the court; or

17.4   a "fault" or "let" has occurred.

18. CONTINUOUS PLAY, MISCONDUCT, PENALTIES

18.1   Play shall be continuous from the first service until the match is concluded, except as allowed in Laws 18.2 and 18.3.

18.2   An interval not exceeding 5 minutes is allowed between the second and third games of all matches in all of the following situations:

    18.2.1   in international competitive events;

    18.2.2   in IBF sanctioned events; and

    18.2.3   in all other matches (unless the National Organization has previously published a decision not to allow such an interval).

18.3   When necessitated by circumstances not within the control of the players, the Umpire may suspend play for such a period as the Umpire may consider necessary. If play be suspended, the existing score shall stand and play be resumed from that point.

18.4   Under no circumstances shall play be suspended to enable a player to recover his strength or wind, or to receive instruction or advice.

18.5.1   Except in the intervals provided in Laws 18.2 and 18.3, no player shall be permitted to receive advice during a match.

18.5.2   Except at the conclusion of a match, no player shall leave the court without the Umpire's consent.

18.6   The Umpire shall be the sole judge of any suspension of play.

18.7 A player shall not:

    18.7.1 deliberately cause suspension of play;

    18.7.2 deliberately interfere with the speed of the shuttle;

    18.7.3 behave in an offensive manner; or

    18.7.4 be guilty of misconduct not otherwise covered by the Laws of Badminton.

18.8 The Umpire shall administer any breach of Law 18.4, 18.5 or 18.7 by:

    18.8.1 issuing a warning to the offending side;

    18.8.2 faulting the offending side, if previously warned; or

    18.8.3 in cases of flagrant offense or persistent offenses, faulting the offending side and reporting the offending side immediately to the Referee, who shall have the power to disqualify.

18.9 Where a Referee has not been appointed, the responsible official shall have the power to disqualify.

19. OFFICIALS AND APPEALS

19.1 The Referee is in overall charge of the tournament or event of which a match forms part.

19.2 The Umpire, where appointed, is in charge of the match, the court and its immediate surrounds. The Umpire shall report to the Referee. In the absence of a Referee, the Umpire shall report instead to the responsible official.

19.3 The Service Judge shall call service faults made by the server should they occur (Law 11).

19.4 A Line Judge shall indicate whether a shuttle is "in" or "out."

An Umpire shall:

19.5 uphold and enforce the Laws of Badminton and, especially call a "fault" or "let" should either occur, without appeal being made by the players;

19.6 give a decision on any appeal regarding a point of dispute, if made before the next service is delivered;

19.7 ensure players and spectators are kept informed of the progress of the match;

19.8 appoint or remove Line Judges or a Service Judge in consultation with the Referee;

19.9 not overrule the decisions of Line Judges and the Service Judge on points of fact;

19.10.1 where another court official is not appointed, arrange for their duties to be carried out;

19.10.2 where an appointed official is unsighted, carry out the official's duties or play a "let";

19.11 decide upon any suspension of play;

19.12 record and report to the Referee all matters in relation to Law 18; and

19.13 Take to the Referee all unsatisfied appeals on questions of Law only.

    (Such appeals must be made before the next service is delivered, or, if at the end of a game, before the side that appeals has left the court.)

Glossary of Badminton Terms

Alley: The 1½-foot-wide area on each side of the court that is used for doubles.

Back alley: The area between the doubles' long service line and the back baseline.

Back court: Approximately the back third of the court.

Backhand: A stroke made on the nonracket side of the body.

Base: *See* Home base. Also the cork part of the shuttle in which the feathers are attached.

Baseline: The back boundary line of the court.

Bird: Another name for shuttlecock or shuttle.

Block: A soft shot, used primarily against a smash, in which there is no backswing or follow-through.

Carry: Called when the shuttle stays on the racket during a stroke. It is legal if the racket follows the intended line of flight. Also called *throw*.

Centerline: The line parallel with the sidelines, separating the service courts.

Clear: A high shot that goes over your opponent's head and lands close to the backline. Also called *lob*.

Combination doubles formation: A strategy in which the partners play both up and back and side by side.

Crosscourt: A shot hit diagonally into the opposite court.

Dab: A blocking action for a shot. Also called *push*.

Double hit: An illegal shot in which the racket contacts the shuttle in one swing.

Doubles service court: The short, wide area (13 feet by 10 feet) to which the server must serve.

Down-the-line shot: A shot hit straight ahead, usually down the sideline.

Dribble: *See* Hairpin drop shot.

Drive: A hard-driven stroke that clears the net but does not go high enough for your opponent to smash.

Drive serve: A hard serve similar to the drive shot. It is used most often in doubles games, with a server serving from the right court to the backhand side of a right-handed player.

Drop: A shot that just clears the net, then falls close to it.

Face: The wide part of the racket—the part with the strings.

Fault: Any infraction of the rules. It results in the loss of serve or in a point for the server.

First serve: A term used in doubles to indicate that the person serving is the first server of the inning.

Flick: A quick wrist action that speeds the flight of the shuttle.

Foot fault: Called when the server's feet are out of the proper service court or when they leave the floor during a serve.

Forecourt: The area near the net—approximately between the net and the short service line.

Forehand: Any stroke made on the racket side of the body.

Game point: The point that ends the game.

Hairpin drop shot: A soft shot made from close to the net and low, just clearing the net and then dropping nearly straight down.

Half-court shot: A low shot that lands at approximately midcourt. It is used most often in doubles against teams playing in an up-and-back alignment.

Hand in: The term used to indicate that the server retains the serve.

Hand out or **one hand down:** The term used in doubles when one player has lost service.

Home base: The position in the center of the court from which the player can best play any shot hit by the opponent.

IBF: The International Badminton Federation—the world governing body.

Inning: The period of time during which a singles player or a doubles team is serving.

Kill: A fast, downward return, such as a smash, which should end the point.

Let: Called when play is stopped because of some outside interference. The point is then replayed.

Lob: *See* Clear.

Long serve: A high serve landing near the back line of the receiver.

Love: A term sometimes used to indicate that the score is zero.

Match: A series of games. The winner must win two out of three games or three out of five to win the match.

Match point: The point that, if won, will win the game.

Midcourt: The middle third of the court, between the net and the baseline.

Net shot: A shot executed in the forecourt that barely clears the top of the net.

Offense: The team or player that is hitting downward returns or forcing the opponent to lift the shuttle in the return.

Overhead: The arm action used to hit a shuttle when it is above one's head.

Placement: Controlling where a shot will land. Good placement directs a shot to an area of the court from which the opponent will find it difficult to make an effective return.

Pronation: The inward rotation of the wrist and forearm used for all forehand strokes that require power.

Put the bird on the floor: End the rally with a kill or a well-hit place where the opponents cannot get a racket on the bird.

Racket: The implement used to hit the shuttle.

Racket foot: The foot on the racket side of the body. It will be forward on underhand strokes.

Rally: A period of hitting the shuttle back and forth over the net—either during practice or during a game.

Ready position: The balanced position that a player assumes to be ready to move in any direction. The weight is on the balls of the feet, knees bent, and the torso leans forward.

Receiver: The player to whom the shuttle is served.

Round-the-head shot: An overhead stroke used when hitting a forehand-like overhead stroke that is on the backhand side of the body.

Rush the serve: A tactic used mostly in doubles by the receiver to quickly attack a low serve.

Scissors: The changing of position of the feet taken during a shot so that the hitter can get to the home-base area more quickly.

Second serve: In doubles, the term indicates that one partner has lost the serve and the other partner is serving.

Server: The player who starts the play.

Setting: Making the choice as to how many more points to play when the score is tied one or two points before the game should be over, such as at 13 or 14 in a 15-point game.

Setup: A shot that gives the opponent an easy chance to win the rally.

Short serve: A serve that clears the net low and lands just beyond the service line. It is used primarily in doubles play.

Shuttlecock or **shuttle**: The feathered cork or plastic missile that is hit in the game of badminton.

Side by side: A defensive formation used in doubles, in which each partner is responsible for one side of the court.

Side out: When the individual or team loses the serve and the other team gets its chance to serve.

Smash: A hard overhead stroke hit sharply downward. It is the major attacking stroke in badminton.

Supination: The outward rotation of the wrist and forearm used for backhand strokes.

T: The intersection of the middle service and short service lines.

Underhand: The stroke used when the shuttle is hit below shoulder level.

Unsight: An illegal position taken by the server's partner so that the receiver cannot see the serve as it is hit.

Up and back: An offensive formation used almost exclusively in mixed doubles, in which the front player is responsible for the forecourt and the partner for the backcourt.

Index

Intensity of exercise, 83, 90
Iron, 81–82

Jacobs, S. J., 16

Karvonen formula, 85
Kerner, A., 16
Kilocalorie, 76, 89

Laws of badminton, 13–16
Left-handed players, 18, 62
Long and short game, 46
Low, backhand serve, 35
Low, short serve, 30, 32

Macronutrients, 76, 89
Magnesium, 82
McHugh, M.P., 16
Micronutrients, 76, 89
Minerals, 79, 81–82, 89, 90
Mixed doubles, 72-74
Muscular endurance, 83

National Badminton Association of
    America, 3
National Cancer Institute, 81
Net, 15
Net player, mixed doubles, 74
Nutrition, 76, 89–90

O'Connor, B., 16
Offensive play(er), 6
    in doubles, 67, 69–70
    in singles, 64
Olympic medal sport, 3
One hand down, 14
Osteoporosis, 82
Overhead clear
    backhand, 47
    forehand, 45–46
Overhead strokes, 44, 46, 54
Overload principle, 83, 90

Phytochemicals, 82, 90
Popularity of badminton, 2, 3
Posture, 86
Protein, 76–78, 89
Pulse rate
    monitoring, 83
    target, 84, 90
Push
    return, 38, 66, 73
    shot, 52

Racket, 6
    foot, 24
    grips, 6, 18–20
    during serve, 28
Rally, 42, 44
    doubles, 67, 69
    singles, 64
Rally ready, 21
Ready position, 26
    rally-, 21
    for return of service, 21–22
Returns
    attacking clear, 36
    clear, 35–36, 38
    doubles, 38–40, 66
    drop, 36, 37, 66
    half-court, 38, 67
    hard drive, 38
    mixed doubles, 72
    push, 38
    service, 20, 35, 63
    singles, 35–37, 63–64
Rotator cuff muscles, 88
Round-the-head-shot, 54
Rules of badminton. *See* Laws of
    badminton

Score/scoring, 12, 13, 41–42
Serve/serving, 13–14, 28
    backhand, 32, 34, 35
    doubles, 13, 14, 41, 42, 66, 74
    drive, 32, 66
    faults, 16, 30
    flick, 32, 33, 63, 66, 72, 73
    high, deep, 28–30
    illegal, 15
    low, short, 30–31, 32, 66, 72
    mixed doubles, 72
    and scoring, 41–42
    tossing for, 13
Server, 8, 14–15, 41
Service
    aces, 44
    court, 8, 13, 28
    line, 8, 13
    returns, 20, 27, 35
Shadow practice, 25
Shoes, 8
Shuttle/shuttlecock, 3, 6, 7, 28, 46
    during serve, 28, 30, 32
    speed of, 2, 33
Shuttle runs, 25
Side-by-side alignment, 67, 68, 70, 74

Singles, 13
    defending against smash in, 58
    home base for, 22
    rally, 64
    returns, 35–37
    serves, 28, 41, 42, 63
    strategy, 53–65, 74
    strokes, 45, 47
    women's, 13
Smash, 12, 21, 36, 48–49, 62, 74
    blocking, 58, 59
    defending, 58, 60, 64
    in doubles, 70
    half-, 50
    in singles, 63, 64, 65
Sportsmanship, 12, 16
Strategy
    basic, 62, 74
    deception as, 62, 66
    defensive, 64, 67
    doubles, 66, 70, 74
    mixed doubles, 72–74
    singles, 63-65, 74
Strength training, 85–88, 90
    abdominal, 85–86
Stretching, 16
Strings, racket, 6
Strokes, overhead, 44, 46, 54

Thomas Cup, 3
Tossing for serve, 13
Triglycerides, 80
Two hands down, 14, 41

Uber Cup, 3
Underhand shots, 44, 60
    clear, 57
    drop, 57, 58
    forehand clear, 56
United States Badminton
    Association, 4
Up-and-back alignment, 69, 70,
    71, 74

Visualization, 88–89
Vitamins, 78, 79, 81, 82, 89, 90

Warm-up, 15–16
    strategy of, 62
Wedge formation, 73, 74
Western grip, 20
Women's singles, 13
Wrist, exercises for, 87–88